MOUSE HEPATIC NEOPLASIA

MOUSE HEPATIC NEOPLASIA

Proceedings of a Workshop held at the H.T.S.
Management Centre, Lane End, High Wycombe (Great Britain)

12–17 May 1974

edited by

W. H. BUTLER, M.B. BS., M.R.C. Path.

Toxicology Unit, M.R.C. Laboratories
Woodmansterne Road
Surrey (Great Britain)

and

P. M. NEWBERNE, D.V.M., Ph. D.

Department of Nutrition and Food Science
Massachusetts Institute of Technology
Cambridge, Mass. 02139 (U.S.A.)

ELSEVIER SCIENTIFIC PUBLISHING COMPANY
AMSTERDAM — OXFORD — NEW YORK
1975

ELSEVIER SCIENTIFIC PUBLISHING COMPANY
335 JAN VAN GALENSTRAAT
P.O. BOX 211, AMSTERDAM, THE NETHERLANDS

AMERICAN ELSEVIER PUBLISHING COMPANY, INC.
52 VANDERBILT AVENUE
NEW YORK, NEW YORK 10017 (U.S.A.)

Library of Congress Cataloging in Publication Data
Main entry under title:

Mouse hepatic neoplasia.

    Includes bibliographical references and index.
    1. Carcinogenesis--Congresses. 2. Liver--Tumors--
Congresses. 3. Oncology, Experimental--Congresses.
4. Mice--Diseases--Congresses. I. Butler, W. H.
II. Newberne, Paul Medford, 1920-   [DNLM:
1. Liver neoplasms--Congresses. 2. Liver neoplasms--
Chemically induced--Congresses. WI735 M932 1974]
RC268.5.M68   616.9'94'36   74-29677
ISBN 0-444-41360-X (New York)

WITH 90 ILLUSTRATIONS AND 47 TABLES

PRINTED IN THE NETHERLANDS

PARTICIPANTS

W. H. Butler, Chairman — MRC Toxicology Unit, Medical Research Council Laboratories, Woodmansterne Road, Carshalton, Surrey (Great Britain)

M. Gellatly — Unilever Research Laboratory, Colworth House, Sharnbrook, Bedford (Great Britain)

P. Grasso — B.I.B.R.A., Woodmansterne Road, Carshalton, Surrey (Great Britain)

H. C. Grice — Food and Drug Directorate, Tunney's Pastures, Ottawa (Canada)

C. F. Hollander — Institute for Experimental Gerontology, 151 Lange Kleiweg, Rijswijk (Z.H.) (The Netherlands)

Glenys Jones — MRC Toxicology Unit, Medical Research Council Laboratories, Woodmansterne Road, Carshalton, Surrey (Great Britain)

G. L. Laqueur — Laboratory of Experimental Pathology, Institute of Arthritis and Metabolic Diseases, Department of Health, Education and Welfare, Public Health Service, Bethesda, Md. 20014 (U.S.A.)

J. W. Newberne — Merrell-National Laboratories, Division of Richardson-Merrell Inc., Cincinnati, Ohio 45215 (U.S.A.)

P. M. Newberne, Chairman — Massachusetts Institute of Technology, Department of Nutrition and Food Science, Room E18-611, Cambridge, Mass. 02139 (U.S.A.)

M. D. Reuber — 11014 Swansfield Road, Columbia, Md. 21044 (U.S.A.)

F. J. C. Roe — 4, Kings Road, Wimbledon, London, SW19 8QN (Great Britain)

Adrianne Rogers — Massachusetts Institute of Technology, Department of Nutrition and Food Science, Room E18-615, Cambridge, Mass. 02139 (U.S.A.)

S. Takayama — Department of Experimental Pathology, Cancer Institute, Japanese Foundation for Cancer Research, Kami-Ikebukuro, Tashima-ku, 170, Tokyo (Japan)

E. Thorpe — Shell Research Limited, Tunstall Laboratories, Sittingbourne, Kent (Great Britain)

OBSERVERS

K. Dix — Shell Research Ltd., Tunstall Laboratories, Sittingbourne, Kent (Great Britain)

G. Edwards — RHM Research Limited, The Lord Rank Research Centre, Lincoln Road, High Wycombe, Bucks. HP1Z 3QR (Great Britain)

P. Hague — Unilever Research Laboratory, Colworth House, Sharnbrook, Bedford (Great Britain)

A. Kemp — Fisons Ltd., Toxicology Department, Chesterford Park Research Station, Saffron Walden, Essex (Great Britain)

B. Leonard — I.C.I. Ltd., Pharmaceuticals Division, Mereside Alderley Park, Macclesfield, Cheshire SK10 4TG (Great Britain)

J. May — RHM Research Limited, The Lord Rank Research Centre, Lincoln Road, High Wycombe, Bucks. HP1Z 3QR (Great Britain)

D. N. Noakes — Fisons Ltd., Agrochemical Division, Chesterford Park Research Station, Saffron Walden, Essex (Great Britain)

J. Offer — Huntingdon Research Centre, Huntingdon, PE18 6ES (Great Britain)

J. McL. Philp — Environmental Safety Officer, Unilever Research, P.O. Box 68, Unilever House, London, EC4P 4BQ (Great Britain)

D. E. Prentice — Huntingdon Research Centre, Huntingdon, PE18 6ES (Great Britain)

I. F. H. Purchase — I.C.I. Limited, Central Toxicology Laboratory, Alderley Park, Nr. Macclesfield, Cheshire, SK10 4TG (Great Britain)

D. Stevenson — Shell Research Limited, Tunstall Laboratories, Sittingbourne, Kent (Great Britain)

G. Williams — The Boots Company Limited, Pharmaceutical Research, Pennyfoot Street, Nottingham, MG2 3AA (Great Britain)

Acknowledgements

We would like to thank the following Companies for the financial support which made the workshop possible.

I.C.I. Pharmaceutical Division,

Shell Research Ltd.,

Unilever Research,

R.H.M. Research Ltd.,

The Boots Company Ltd.,

Fisons Ltd., Agrochemical Division,

Huntingdon Research Centre.

We would also like to thank the participants who prepared working papers and the discussants for their contributions. Such a meeting requires an enormous amount of work both in preparing the working papers and recording and editing the discussions. For this we are indebted to the help of Dr. Glenys Jones and Dr. Adrianne Rogers without whom it would have been impossible to hold and report the workshop.

Abbreviations

2-AAF, 2-acetylaminofluorene
ADAB, 4-amino-2,3-dimethylazobenzene
o-AT, aminoazotoluene
B(a)A, benz(a)anthracene
BCHE, bichloromethylether
BHC, benzenehexachloride
CMME, chloromethyl-methylether
DAB, 4-dimethylazobenzene
DEN, diethylnitrosamine
DMBA, 7,12-dimethyl(a)anthracene; 9,10-dimethyl-1,2-benzanthracene
DMN, dimethylnitrosamine
2,7-FAA, N,N'-2,7-fluorenylenebisacetamide
GF mice, germ-free mice
NBU, N-nitrosobutylurea
N-OH-FAA, N-hydroxy-N-fluoren-2-yl acetamide
OH-AAF, OH-acetylaminofluorene
SER, smooth endothelial reticulum
SP diet, stock pelleted diet
SPF mice, specific pathogen-free (inbred) mice
SSP diet, semisynthetic diet

Preface

In recent years the mouse has been used in increasing numbers both in basic cancer research and safety evaluation of chemicals for use as drugs, food additives and pesticides. One of the commonest sites of induction of neoplasia in the mouse is the liver. In reviewing the literature and taking note of international controversy and discussion on the nature of mouse liver lesions it became evident that there is widespread divergence of opinion on both the diagnosis of such lesions and their significance. The published work is spread widely and thinly throughout the literature.

In view of this, we considered it important to bring together an international group of pathologists who had not only a divergence of opinion but also divergent experience. We considered it important to keep the group small in order to facilitate discussion which was recorded and included in each chapter.

The choice of participants at the workshop was entirely at the discretion of the editors and any opinions expressed by the participants should be considered to be the opinions of the individuals and not of any organization. The Companies supporting this workshop were invited to send two observers.

High Wycombe   W. H. Butler
May 1974   P. M. Newberne

Contents

Chapter 1

Introduction

W. H. BUTLER and P. M. NEWBERNE

MRC Toxicology Unit, Medical Research Council Laboratories,
Woodmansterne Road, Carshalton, Surrey (Great Britain),
and Massachusetts Institute of Technology,
Department of Nutrition and Food Science,
Room E18-611, Cambridge, Mass. 02139 (U.S.A.)

The induction of hepatic neoplasia in the mouse has been used for many years in studies of the biology of neoplasia. The mouse has also been used extensively in safety evaluation of new compounds. In these situations the interpretation of the experimental test depends upon the assessment of the pathology of the lesions induced. At the I.A.R.C. Working Conference on Liver Cancer held at the Chester Beatty Research Institute in 1969 the problem of interpretation of focal proliferative lesions of the mouse liver was discussed and it was apparent that there was little agreement or uniformity in the diagnosis of such lesions. The interpretation of the nature of a single lesion varied from hyperplasia to malignant neoplasia in the absence of invasion and metastases. In the absence of factual information on the biological behaviour of the lesions, these opinions are based upon the experience of the individual pathologists. Inevitably, this experience is variable.

The divergence of opinions was clearly demonstrated in two exercises undertaken to assess the degree of variation of opinion. In an unpublished study, opinions were obtained on a selection of ten lesions induced in mouse liver by a pesticide. In no case was there unanimity of opinion and of the ten pathologists consulted, seven attended the present workshop. A further study, presented by Dr. Takayama at this workshop, was undertaken in Japan. A series of 43 cases was submitted to 15 pathologists and again there was no unanimity of opinion. Also, there was a lack of consistency of individual opinions. While in many cases there was a measure of agreement, in others wide variation was apparent. This is best illustrated in the case shown in Fig. 1, which was classified as hyperplasia by Pathologist No. 10 and malignant neoplasia by Pathologist No. 1. The lesion illustrated in Fig. 2 was classified as malignant by Pathologist No. 10 and hyperplasia by Pathologist No. 1. The entire group agreed that the lesion represented in Fig. 3 was hyperplasia (Case 25) and in Fig. 4 was malignant neoplasia (Case 23). Detailed results of this study are given in Appendix I.

There are possible explanations for these discrepancies resulting from the inevitable disparity of training and experience of the pathologists. However, whatever the cause of the disparity, it is evidently a widespread phenomenon. If the assessment of an

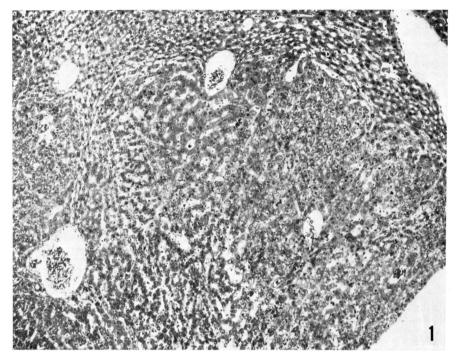

Fig. 1. Photomicrograph of lesion No. 7 diagnosed as liver cell carcinoma by pathologist 1 and hyperplastic nodule by pathologist 10. H and E. ×60.

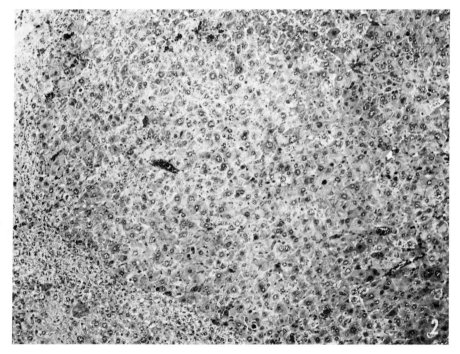

Fig. 2. Photomicrograph of lesion No. 24 diagnosed as hyperplastic nodule by pathologist 1 and liver cell carcinoma by pathologist 10. H and E. ×140.

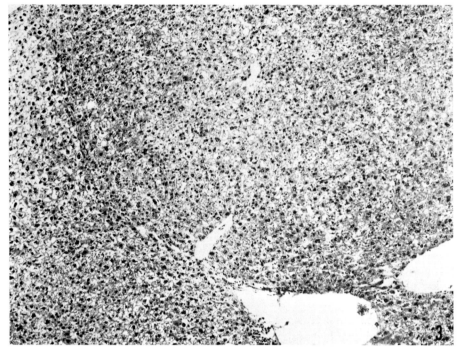

Fig. 3. Photomicrograph of lesion No. 25 diagnosed as hyperplastic nodule by all pathologists. H and E. ×60.

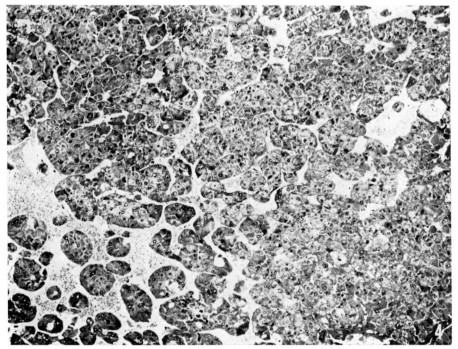

Fig. 4. Photomicrograph of lesion No. 23 diagnosed as liver cell carcinoma by all pathologists. H and E. ×140.

experiment or test is based on the pathological interpretations of induced lesions, any disagreement in this interpretation obviously limits the usefulness of the system.

In any discussion of pathology, it is important to agree on the terminology to be used. For this we suggest following the I.A.R.C. Working Conference (1971).

A. Neoplasm arising from liver parenchymal cells:
   Benign—liver cell adenoma
   Malignant—hepatocellular carcinoma
B. Neoplasm arising from the intrahepatic biliary system:
   Benign—bile duct adenoma or cholangioma
   Malignant—cholangiocarcinoma
C. Neoplasm arising from vascular elements:
   Benign—haemangioendothelioma
   Malignant—angiosarcoma

Nodular hyperplasia is considered to be a focal, non-neoplastic proliferation of hepatic parenchymal cells in excess of the norm. We would also agree with the recommendation of the Working Conference that the term "hepatoma" be abandoned in view of the different connotation to those in the human diagnostic field and the experimental field.

In absolute terms, the presence of invasion or metastases enables the pathologist to make the definitive diagnosis of malignant neoplasia. The problems arise in the assessment of lesions in the absence of these criteria and will be discussed in the present workshop.

The practical problems do not cease even when there is agreement on the pathology of the lesion. Evaluation of safety of a compound requires that an assessment of the significance of any pathological change be made. As in the interpretation of pathology there are marked differences of opinions on this subject. Again referring to the I.A.R.C. Working Conference on Liver Cancer "their significance in toxicological work is uncertain".

The problem of the significance of many lesions has been discussed by GRASSO AND CRAMPTON (1972) who suggested that the interpretation of lesions such as those in the mouse liver must be made with extreme caution. The disparity of opinion as to the significance and its extrapolation to man is well illustrated in public hearings in the U.S.A. concerning the registration of DDT. Various opinions were expressed of the pathological interpretation of the liver lesions and their significance. One body of opinion was that the induction of nodules in the mouse liver, which were considered to be malignant, provided definitive evidence of the carcinogenicity of DDT and hence represented a high risk to man. Other opinions expressed the view that the malignant nature of the lesions had not been demonstrated and it was not possible to extrapolate the data to man in any meaningful way.

Further it has been suggested that large scale tests using the mouse be undertaken in order to demonstrate weakly active carcinogens and obtain statistically significant results. It is obviously important that the pathological lesions seen in the liver be interpretable without equivocation.

We have endeavoured in the present workshop to gather together in one place the available data on mouse hepatic neoplasia to enable the practising pathologist to assess the information. Further, we have considered the problem of the biological significance of lesions produced in mouse liver and discussed the extrapolation of them to questions of safety evaluation of chemicals for human use. We do not consider that at present it is possible to give definitive answers to many of the problems. However, it is important that a rational assessment of the pathology be made prior to an interpretation of any significance to man.

REFERENCES

GRASSO, P., AND CRAMPTON, R. (1972) The value of the mouse in carcinogenicity testing. *Food Cosmet. Toxicol.*, 10: 418.
Liver Cancer, 1971, I.A.R.C. Scientific Publications No. 1. International Agency for Research on Cancer, Lyon (France).

Chapter 2

Embryology and Ageing Effects

C. F. HOLLANDER

*Institute for Experimental Gerontology TNO,
Rijswijk—ZH (The Netherlands)*

In the mouse, as in other mammalian species, the liver develops from a ventral outgrowth of the gut endoderm. It is not my intention to describe in detail the complete embryology of the mouse liver, but just to bring to your attention those features which might be relevant to this meeting.

The earliest recognizable liver parenchyma is found in the mouse at day 9 post coitum and consists of buds of epithelial cords embedded in splanchnic mesoderm (Fig. 1) (BERKVENS, 1974). At day 10, epithelial cords are seen which are separated by large cystic spaces in which haemopoiesis takes place (Fig. 2). During the following days, further development takes place and, at day 16, epithelial cords covered by lining endothelium of the broad sinusoids can hardly be recognized. This is due to the very active haemopoiesis which takes place in the liver (Fig. 3). It should be mentioned that, up to this time, the liver is the main haemopoietic organ. In most inbred mouse strains, the main activity of haemopoiesis has shifted to the bone marrow and the spleen at day 7 after birth, and only a few minor foci of haemopoiesis can be found in the liver (Figs. 4 and 5). In adult and aged mice, foci of extramedullary haemopoiesis can be found in the sinusoids (Fig. 6), around the central vein (Fig. 7) or in the reticular tissue of the interlobular septa (DUNN, 1954). There are indications that the liver retains its capacity for extramedullary haemopoiesis during the entire lifespan of the mouse (B. LÖWENBERG, personal communication). Extramedullary haemopoiesis must be differentiated from invasion of the liver by erythroblastosis due to the Rauscher virus, lymphosarcoma, or reticulum cell sarcoma.

The liver occupies the anterior third of the abdominal cavity and consists of four main lobes which are joined dorsally. These are: the large median lobe, subdivided into left and right portions by a deep bifurcation; the undivided left lateral lobe; the right lateral lobe, divided horizontally into anterior and posterior portions; and a caudal lobe consisting of two leaf-shaped lobes dorsal and ventral to the oesophagus at the lesser curvature of the stomach. Numerous patterns of lobulation have been described. However, the above-mentioned is most commonly observed. The circulation of blood in the liver is provided by interlobular branches of the hepatic artery and the hepatic portal vein which open into the sinusoids separating cords of liver cells. The sinusoids mainly communicate with central veins which are tributaries of hepatic veins. The gall bladder is located at the base of the deep bifurcation of the

8

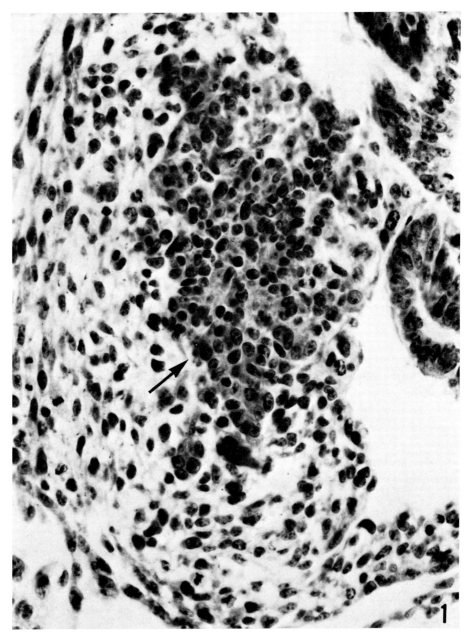

Fig. 1. Earliest recognizable liver anlage (arrow) in a Swiss mouse (CD-Charles River) embryo at day 9 post coitum (HPS, ×500).

median lobe near the point of origin of the falciform ligament. The hepatic duct from the liver and the cystic duct from the gall bladder unite to form the common bile duct. A good description of the anatomy and histology of the mouse liver is given by HUMMEL *et al.* (1966).

Mice and rats, which have a relatively short life-span, are traditionally used in the

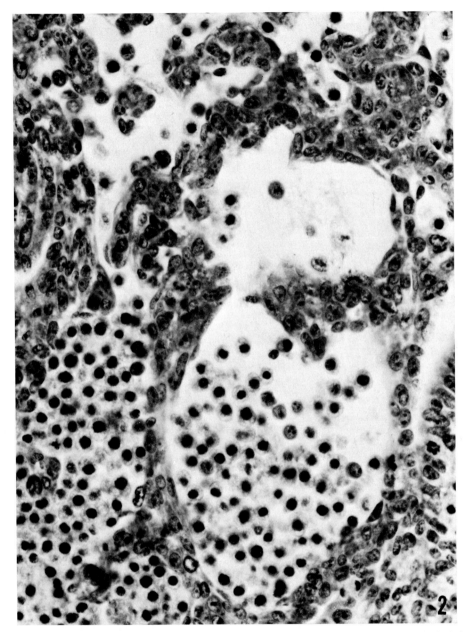

Fig. 2. Liver of a Swiss mouse (CD-Charles River) day 10 post coitum showing haemopoiesis in cystic like spaces. (HPS, ×500).

laboratory for ageing studies. However, the widely used inbred strains of rodents were developed and selected for cancer research and not primarily for studying the process of ageing (HOLLANDER, 1973). Two strains of the same inbred species may live to the same age and yet show a different slope of mortality curve (Text-fig. 1A). This difference in the slope of the curve can be explained by the different causes of death in the

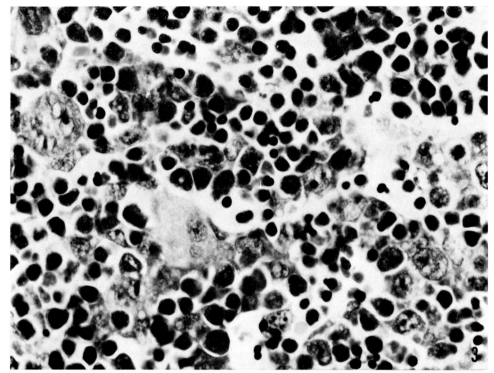

Fig. 3. Liver of a C57BL/KaLwRij mouse day 16 post coitum showing active haemopoiesis. The liver parenchymal cells can be hardly recognized. (HPS, ×728).

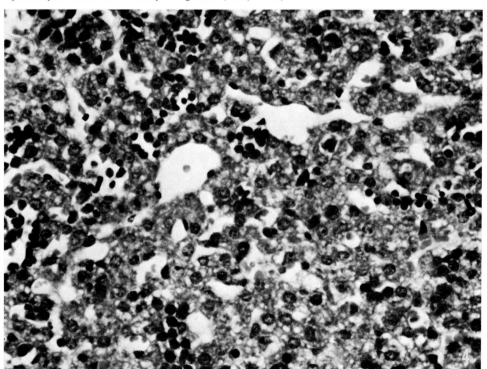

Fig. 4. Liver of a 1-day-old CBA/BrARij mouse still showing numerous foci of haemopoiesis. (HPS, ×400).

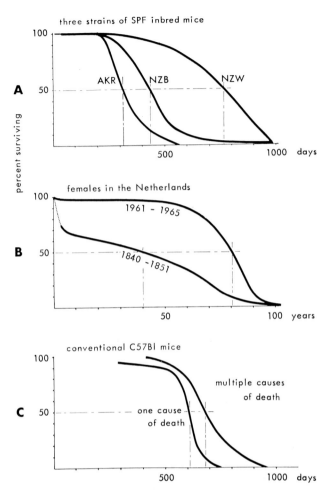

Text-fig. 1. Survival curves of: (A) 3 strains of specific pathogen-free (SPF) inbred mice; (B) female humans in the Netherlands at 2 different time periods; and (C) conventional C57BL mice dying of one cause and multiple causes (see also HOLLANDER, 1973).

NZB mouse and the NZW mouse. In the first strain, the main cause of death is related to haemolytic auto-immune anaemia. In the NZW mouse, as in man, there are multiple causes of death. Furthermore, in the AKR mouse (Text-fig. 1A), the incidence of leukaemia approaches 100% at a relatively young age and this type of cancer severely limits the maximum as well as the medium life-span of the AKR mouse as compared to the NZW mouse. Also, intercurrent infections which become the main cause of death may markedly affect the slope of the mortality curve (Text-fig. 1C). The same holds true for man (Text-fig. 1B). The shift of the survival curve to the right during the period 1960–1965 can be explained by the control of acute infectious diseases, improved medical care, and improved hygienic conditions.

For ageing studies, as in other long-term investigations, the primary requirement of today is for animals of good quality, e.g., SPF and sometimes germ-free (GF) animals. The cost of producing and maintaining such animals is an additional financial

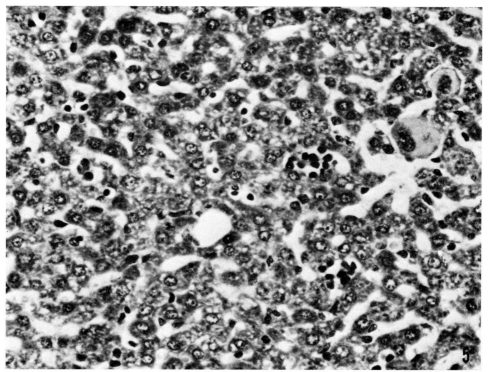

Fig. 5. Liver of a 7-day-old CBA/BrARij mouse showing few foci of haemopoiesis. Note mega-karyocytes in sinusoid. (HPS, ×400).

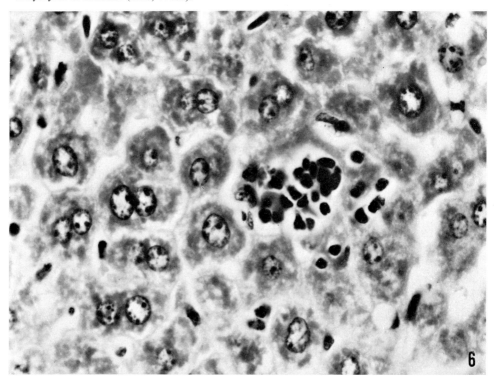

Fig. 6. Liver of a 32-month-old CBA/BrARij mouse with a focus of extramedullary haemopoiesis in a sinusoid. (HPS, ×728).

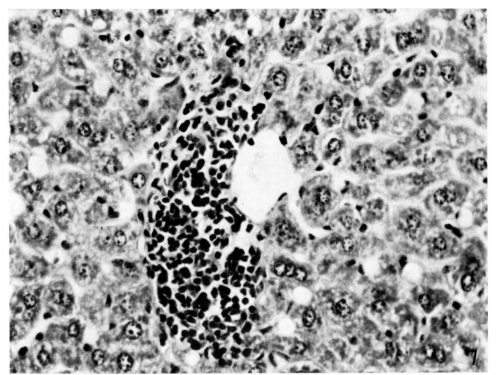

Fig. 7. Liver of the same mouse as Fig. 6 with a focus of extramedullary haemopoiesis next to a central vein. (HPS, ×400).

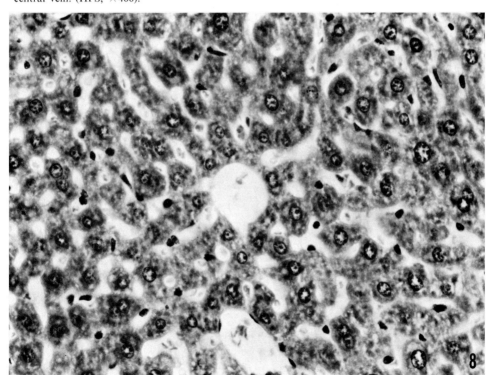

Fig. 8. Liver of a 21-day-old CBA/BrARij mouse without haemopoiesis and already polyploidization of liver cells. (HPS, ×400).

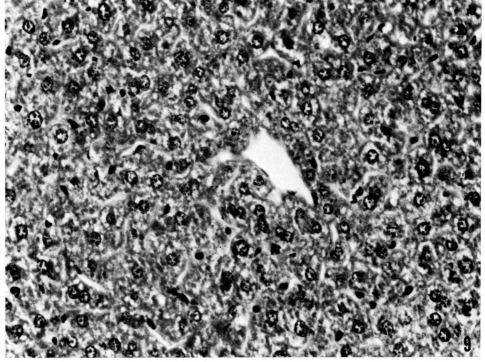

Fig. 9. Liver of a 12-month-old CBA/BrARij mouse. Note slightly more conspicious polyploidization of liver cells. (HPS, ×400).

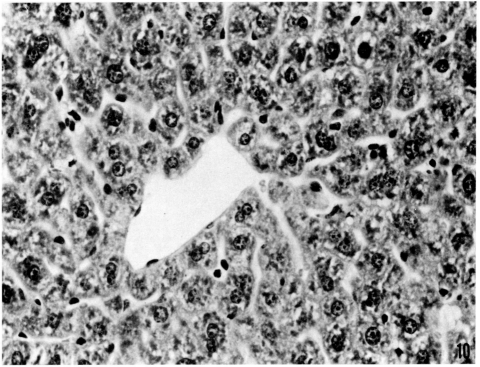

Fig. 10. Liver of a 24-month-old CBA/BrARij mouse. Compare with Figs. 8 and 9 for degree of liver cell polyploidization. (HPS, ×400).

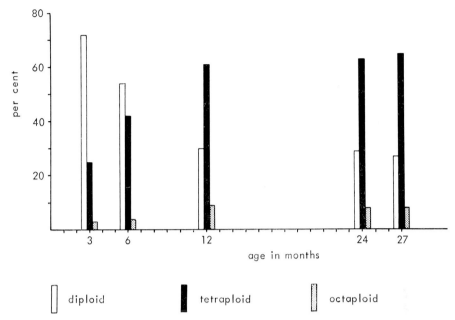

Text-fig. 2. Percentage distribution of mononuclear classes of parenchymal cells isolated from female RU rats of different ages. Each bar represents the mean of two rats in which 2000 nuclei were measured per animal.

burden to the already expensive experiments. Therefore, the animals should be optimally used and adequate information should be given on the animals used. Optimum information can be reached by providing mortality curves combined with morbidity data. Knowing the slope of the mortality curve will enable the reader of scientific publications to draw conclusions on the validity of the term "an old mouse".

WARREN ANDREW (1971), in his monograph on *The Anatomy of Aging in Man and Animals,* has dealt exhaustively with the different aspects of ageing of the liver in mice. Our histological studies confirm the observations made by ANDREW and others that the aged mouse liver does not show characteristic ageing changes as compared to the adult mouse liver. There is no conspicuous fibrosis. In the literature dealing with ageing aspects of the liver in man and animals, one frequently encounters the statement that polyploidy of liver cells is a typical ageing phenomenon. However, studies conducted by DE LEEUW-ISRAEL (1971) and VAN BEZOOIJEN et al. (1972/73, 1974) in our Institute have proven beyond doubt that liver cell polyploidization in the rat occurs early in life and is strain-dependent (Text-fig. 2.3). SWARTZ (1956) has found that the main shift of liver cell polyploidization occurs before puberty in man. Data from the literature (LESHER et al., 1960; EPSTEIN AND GATENS, 1967) indicate that liver cell polyploidization is also not an ageing phenomenon in mice (Figs. 8, 9, 10).

In the aged liver of the mouse, aberrant parenchymal cells with giant nuclei can be observed. ANDREW et al. (1943) were the first to describe intranuclear inclusions in parenchymal cells of senile human as well as mouse livers (Fig. 11). These inclusions seemed to be similar to those described by LEDUC AND WILSON (1959 a,b) after

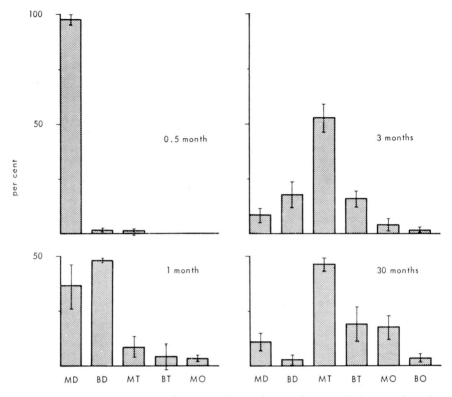

Text-fig. 3. Percentage distribution of nuclear classes of parenchymal cells isolated from female WAG/Rij rats of different ages. Each bar represents the mean of 4 separate experiments. The standard deviation of the mean is indicated by the vertical lines. For each experiment, 200 nuclei were measured. MD, mononuclear diploid; BD, binuclear diploid; MT, mononuclear tetraploid; BT, binuclear tetraploid; MO, mononuclear octaploid; BO, binuclear octaploid.

chemical damage to the mouse liver as well as in some mouse hepatomas. They actually represent invaginations of the nuclear membrane with entrapped masses of cytoplasm (Fig. 12). The same type of inclusions have also been observed in 3-month-old mice after partial hepatectomy and in spontaneous hepatomas (HOLLANDER AND THUNG, 1966). At present, there are no substantial data to prove that the occurrence of these intranuclear inclusions is an expression of ageing of liver cells. However, in the search for these intranuclear inclusions, one is apt to find them more readily in an aged liver.

Unlike the neurons of the brain and the muscle cells of the heart, there is no increasing deposition of lipofuscin pigment in the mouse liver with increasing age. It is observed only in small quantities.

In her thesis on *Ageing Changes in the Rat Liver. An Experimental Study of Hepatocellular Function and Morphology*, DE LEEUW-ISRAEL (1971) has reviewed the literature on functional changes in the liver with age.

The generalized tendency of aged tissues, and in this case the liver, to hyperplasia and neoplasia and the strain dependence is a subject which wil be dealt with in more

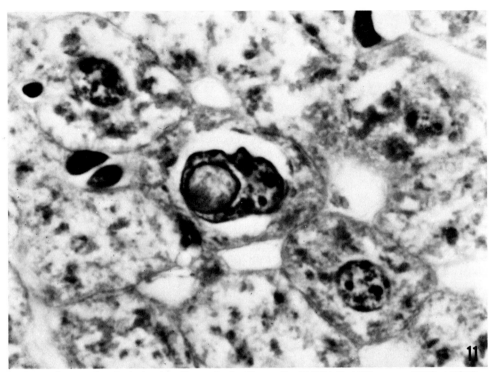

Fig. 11. Intranuclear inclusion in a liver cell of a 23-month-old CBA/BrARij mouse. (HPS, ×1816).

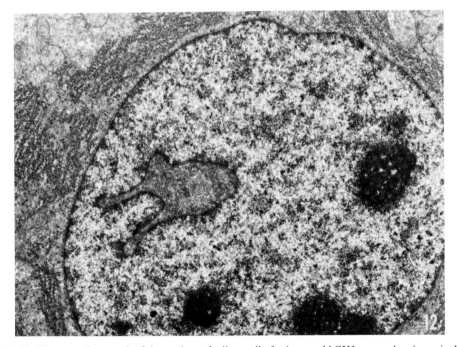

Fig. 12. Electron micrograph of the nucleus of a liver cell of a 1-year-old C3H mouse showing a single cytoplasmic inclusion (×7360).

detail by other speakers at this meeting. These might be the most conspicuous ageing lesions in the mouse liver.

SUMMARY

The embryology and anatomy of the mouse liver is briefly reviewed. No conspicuous ageing changes are observed in the mouse liver except for the generalized tendency of aged tissues to hyperplasia and neoplasia. However, this subject will be dealt with elsewhere at this meeting.

ACKNOWLEDGEMENT

The author gratefully acknowledges the assistance of Drs. C. F. A. van Bezooijen, Miss A. L. Nooteboom and Mr. A. A. Glaudemans, Institute for Experimental Gerontology TNO and Dr. Johanna M. Berkvens, Laboratory of Pathology, National Institute of Public Health, Bilthoven, The Netherlands in the preparation of the manuscript. Dr. Johanna M. Berkvens also supplied the material for Figs. 1 and 2. Dr. W. H. Butler, MRC Toxicology Unit, Carshalton, England, supplied Fig. 12.

REFERENCES

ANDREW, W. (1971) *The Anatomy of Aging in Man and Animals*. Grune and Stratton, New York, pp. 161–171.
ANDREW, W., BROWN, H. M., AND JOHNSON, J. B. (1943) Senile changes in the liver of mouse and man with special reference to the similarity of the nuclear alterations. *Amer. J. Anat.*, 72: 199–221.
BERKVENS, J. M. (1974) Embryology of the mouse. *Biotechniek*, 13: 1–44.
DE LEEUW-ISRAEL, F. R. (1971) *Aging Changes in the Rat Liver. An Experimental Study of Hepatocellular Function and Morphology*. Thesis, University of Leyden. (Available as publication of the Institute for Experimental Gerontology TNO, Rijswijk-ZH, The Netherlands.)
DUNN, T. B. (1954) Normal and pathologic anatomy of the reticular tissue in laboratory mice, with a classification and discussion of neoplasms. *J. Natl. Cancer Inst.*, 14: 1281–1434.
EPSTEIN, C. J. (1967) Cell size, nuclear content, and the development of polyploidy in the mammalian liver. *Proc. Natl. Acad. Sci. (U.S.)*, 57; 327–334.
EPSTEIN, C. J., AND GATENS, E. A. (1967) Nuclear ploidy in mammalian parenchymal liver cells. *Nature*, 214; 1050–1051.
HOLLANDER, C. F. (1973) Animal models for aging and cancer research. *J. Natl. Cancer Inst.*, 51: 3–5.
HOLLANDER, C. F., AND THUNG, P. J. (1966) Relations between regenerative growth and aging in the mouse liver. in LINDOP, P. J., AND SACHER, G. A. (Eds.), *Radiation and Ageing*. Taylor and Francis, London, pp. 3–14.
HUMMEL, K. P., RICHARDSON, F. L., AND FEKETE, E. (1966) Anatomy. in GREEN, E. L. (Ed.), *Biology of the Laboratory Mouse*, 2nd ed. McGraw-Hill, New York, Chapter 13, pp. 280–281.
LEDUC, E. H., AND WILSON, J. W. (1959a) A histochemical study of intranuclear inclusions in mouse liver and hepatoma. *J. Histochem. Cytochem.*, 7: 8–16,
LEDUC, E. H., AND WILSON, J. W. (1959b) An electron microscope study of intranuclear inclusions in mouse liver and hepatoma. *J. biophys. biochem. Cytol.*, 6: 427–430.
LESHER, S., STROUD, A. N., AND BRUES, A. M. (1960) The effects of chronic irradiation on DNA synthesis in regenerating mouse liver. *Cancer Res.*, 20: 1341–1346.

SWARTZ, F. J. (1956) The development in the human liver of multiple desoxyribose nucleic acid (DNA) classes and their relationship to the age of the individual. *Chromosoma*, 8: 53–72.

VAN BEZOOIJEN, C. F. A., DE LEEUW-ISRAEL, F. R., AND HOLLANDER, C. F. (1972/73) On the role of hepatic cell ploidy in changes in liver function with age and following partial hepatectomy. *Mech. Age. Dev.*, 1: 351–356.

VAN BEZOOIJEN, C. F. A., VAN NOORD, M. J., AND KNOOK, D. L. (1974) The viability of parenchymal liver cells isolated from young and old rats. *Mech. Age. Dev.*, 3: 107–119.

DISCUSSION

BUTLER. Does hepatoblastoma correspond to any stage of the development of the liver?

HOLLANDER. Not in my opinion. In the human hepatoblastomas the cells are totally different from those seen in embryonic liver.

GELLATLY. To me it is a hepatic carcinoma of very poor differentiation. The term is seldom used in the literature.

ROE. I would like to ask about Figs. 6 and 7 in which you describe haematopoiesis. Very often there are collections of lymphocyte-like cells around blood vessels and this is frequently referred to as haematopoiesis. Is there any good evidence that this is so?

HOLLANDER. In some cases it is possible to identify haematopoietic cells but in many instances it is doubtful. The differential diagnosis would be: (*1*) tumour, (*2*) haematopoiesis, (*3*) inflammatory reaction. In the cases I have described, there is no destruction of the parenchymal cells, and mitoses may be present in the foci indicating proliferation. Although this is a common finding, I would consider that there is little evidence that in fact these are haematopoietic in nature.

P. M. NEWBERNE. I was interested to see the results of the ploidy changes which seemed to come to an end by twelve months with a plateau. This is contrary to the generally held view.

HOLLANDER. We did not recognise this plateau until we set up a long-term study, in which after one and a half years we found that there was a parallel between the function of the liver, as measured by bromsulphthalein clearance or albumin production, and polyploidy. We found strain differences also. We then asked what is an old animal? For this it is necessary to know the survival data, for the colony to make any interpretations of the findings of polyploidy. These findings may be modified by factors other than age. There is, when looking at Fig. 10 of the working paper, an apparent increased variation in nuclear size in the liver. However, when one studies the ploidy within these livers, there appears to be a plateau at about twelve months, although after this there is some increase of octaploids.

ROE. It is very difficult to know whether any change we see in old mice is related to age as it may just as well be due to a longer experience of the environment. In logic I do not see how you can be sure that anything is primarily due to age.

GRICE. With better management and breeding procedures, the life-span of rats and mice is far beyond that of ten years ago. Most testing procedures in rats last two years and in mice eighteen months. Do you have any information for mice at thirty months of age and would you consider that a carcinogenicity test should go beyond eighteen months in mice?

HOLLANDER. It is obviously very difficult to recommend the duration of a test for carcinogenicity. To be fair one should possibly do the longer term tests. I only see "pathological" ageing and do not really know what "physiological" ageing is.

GELLATLY. I did not look upon this paper as an age-related paper. I look upon it as background pathology. Those of us that have looked at the literature will realize how little attention is paid to the extra-nodular parenchyma of the mouse liver. Many of us have seen changes in ploidy and in binucleate cells but we also see modification of the nuclei, which consists of condensed central nuclear chromatin as well as peripheral chromatin. It always occurs at the periphery of the lobes. We compared two diets, a semi-purified diet and a stock standard diet. We were interested in whether this or any of the background pathological changes correlated with the incidence of nodules on the same diet. The details of our findings are given in my working paper (GELLATLY, Chapter 8).

Chapter 3

Morphology of Spontaneous and Induced Neoplasia

GLENYS JONES AND W. H. BUTLER

MRC Toxicology Unit,
Medical Research Council Laboratories,
Woodmansterne Road,
Carshalton,
Surrey (Great Britain)

INTRODUCTION

Of the many species used in both experimental carcinogenesis and in testing programmes, the mouse is the most common. In spite of this there are relatively few detailed accounts of the morphology of hepatic neoplasia. The commonest hepatic neoplasm observed is derived from the parenchymal cells and is frequently referred to in the literature as "hepatoma" without further designation. The lesions may vary in size from microscopic nodules (CLAPP AND CRAIG, 1967) to large bizarre nodules many cm in diameter (WALKER *et al.*, 1972). The lesions may occur "spontaneously" or may be induced. The best description of both the induced and spontaneous "hepatomas" is that of ANDERVONT AND DUNN (1952). They describe nodules of hepatic parenchymal cells which appear very similar to the non-neoplastic surrounding liver. The surrounding liver was compressed but no invasion or metastasis was seen. The "spontaneous hepatomas" were considered to be indistinguishable from the lesions induced by carbon-tetrachloride (EDWARDS AND DALTON, 1943), *o*-aminoazotoluene (ANDERVONT AND GRADY, 1942) or diethylnitrosamine (CLAPP AND CRAIG, 1967) and phenobarbitone (PERAINO *et al.*, 1973). Similar lesions have been induced in adult mice following neonatal administration of a wide variety of compounds.

Vascular neoplasia is often induced in the mouse liver. This lesion has been reported following *o*-aminoazotoluene (ANDERVONT AND GRADY, 1942) urethane (TRAININ, 1963; KAWAMOTO *et al.*, 1961) and dimethylnitrosamine (DMN) (TAKAYAMA AND OOTA, 1965). Metastases have been described indicating that at least in some instances this is malignant neoplasia.

In the mouse both spontaneous and induced biliary neoplasia are rare. REUBER (1967) and VLAHAKIS AND HESTON (1971) have described spontaneous cholangiomas while TAKAYAMA AND INUI (1967) reported four adenohepatomas. The morphology of these lesions will be described later in this working paper. There is considerable disagreement as to the correct diagnosis of many of the lesions included in this working paper. It is intended that as many as possible of the lesions which have been described as neoplastic will be included without initially giving an opinion as to the nature of the

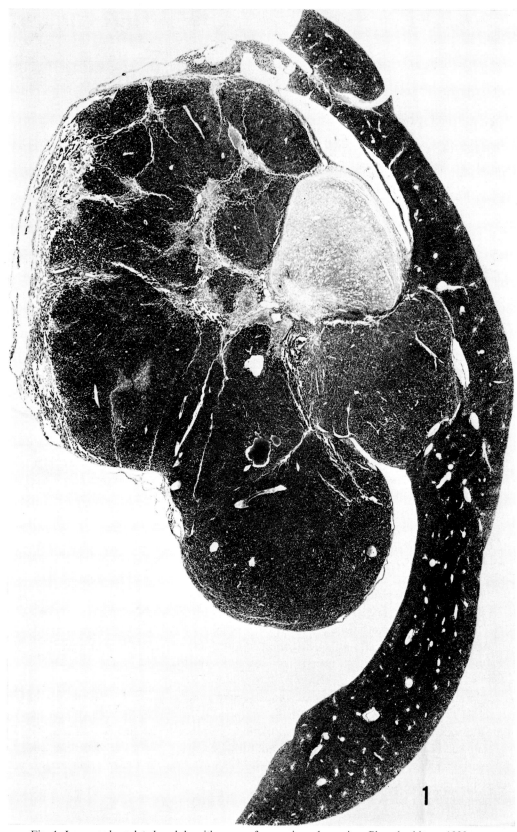

Fig. 1. Large pedunculated nodule with areas of necrosis and scarring. Phenobarbitone 1000 ppm in the diet. H and E × 10.

lesion other than that it is a nodule. In the case of parenchymal cell nodules this will be taken to mean a focal proliferative lesion disturbing the architecture of the liver. The problem of differential diagnosis of these lesions will be considered in the discussion.

For this working paper material has been obtained from many sources. In our own laboratories inbred C3H male mice have been followed for their life span in order to obtain "spontaneous" nodules, which occur in approximately 20% of two-year survivors. C3H male mice have been fed 1000 ppm phenobarbitone continuously. By 70 weeks 74% of the mice developed macroscopic nodules which were studied either by conventional histology, or were fixed for electron microscopy. Of the latter 6 were perfused fixed for large-area plastic sectioning. Other tissues were taken for routine histology, and the lungs from 23 treated and 4 control mice, all with nodules, were serial-sectioned in 100 μ steps and examined for the presence of metastases. Fifty C3H male mice were fed 25 ppm DMN continuously from weaning. The longest survival was 40 weeks and 8 mice were found to have nodular vascular liver lesions. No animal had a parenchymal cell nodule. These animals were examined by routine histology.

In addition extensive use has been made of materials supplied by Dr. E. Thorpe, Tunstall Laboratory, Shell Research Limited. This material included spontaneous nodules as well as lesions induced by DDT, dieldrin and scarlet red. Further material from mice treated with DDT (L. Tomatis, IARC, Lyon), DMN (L. den Engelse, C. F. Hollander and W. Mindorp, Institute of Gerontology, Rijswijk, Z.H.) and acetylaminofluorene (P. M. Newberne, Massachusetts Institute of Technology) has been studied. The spontaneous cholangioma was supplied by Dr. M. D. Reuber (University of Maryland).

Mouse liver tumours can be divided into four main groups.

(1) Parenchymal. The multiple nodular lesions found in control mice and induced by compounds, such as DDT, dieldrin and phenobarbitone, acetylaminofluorene and nitrosamines.

(2) Vascular. Spontaneously occurring vascular nodules, haemangioendothelioma and haemangiosarcoma induced by compounds such as DMN.

(3) Tumours arising from the bile duct. Cholangioma.

(4) Others, e.g. lymphoreticular lesions.

The parenchymal cell nodules. The nodules occurring in control mice and mice undergoing long-term feeding with a variety of compounds including DDT, phenobarbitone, dieldrin, scarlet red, have been described as having a similar morphology. The incidence of these nodules in control mice varies according to strain and sex and is dis-

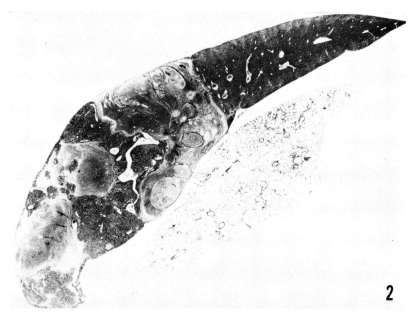

Fig. 2. Extensive haemorrhage and necrosis within liver nodules. Phenobarbitone 1000 ppm in diet. H and E×5.6.

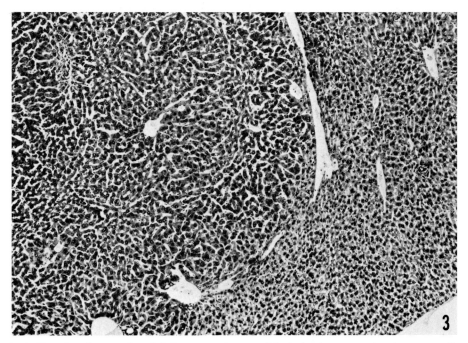

Fig. 3. The edge of a type A nodule in a control mouse. The lesion is compressing the surrounding normal liver and the vessels of the portal tract are stretched around its periphery. Note the regular arrangement of the trabeculae in the nodule and the difficulty of distinguishing it from the normal liver. H and E×56.

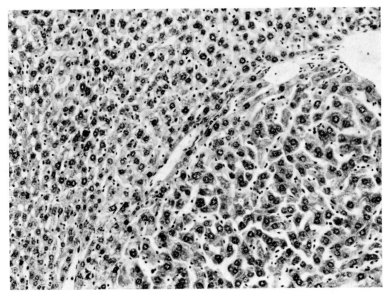

Fig. 4. High power photomicrograph of the edge of the nodule illustrated in Fig. 3. H and E × 130.

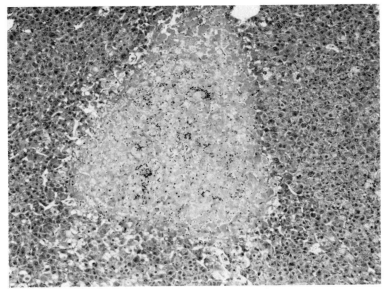

Fig. 5. A small infarct in a type A nodule induced by DDT. H and E × 56. (E. THORPE)

cussed by Dr. P. GRASSO (Chapter 6). Untreated C3H and CF1 male mice have a reported incidence up to 30 %, female mice 5 %. Long-term feeding of dieldrin 10 ppm increases this to 90 % (WALKER *et al.*, 1972) and phenobarbitone 500 ppm to 90 % (THORPE AND WALKER, 1973).

The nodules vary in size from 1 to 2 mm to several cm diameter (Fig. 1). Multiple lesions are found in a single liver and occur in all lobes. They vary in colour from white to reddish brown and may contain cystic, haemorrhagic and infarcted areas (Fig. 2). Large lobulated masses cause abdominal distension of the mice.

WALKER *et al.* (1972) classify these lesions into two histological types. *Type A*, simple nodular growth of liver parenchymal cells. Solid cords of closely packed cells with staining and morphology little different from the rest of the non-nodular parenchyma. Mitotic activity is evident but sparse. There is compression of the surrounding liver cells but no evidence of a capsule. Lesions may be single or multiple. No fibrosis is seen in the liver. *Type B*, nodules of liver parenchymal cells showing areas of papilliform and adenoid growth. Cells are in confluent sheets with areas of necrosis. The vascular spaces are wide and irregular. Nuclear abnormalities are common with many inclusions, hyperchromasia and many mitoses. Hydropic fatty change and hyalin droplet formation are common.

This classification is used in this review but it must be stressed that these are not definite divisions and many lesions contain areas of both A and B morphology. The small 2-mm diam. lesions are invariably type A, but the larger nodules cannot be classified by size. Single livers can contain multiple areas of A and B nodules. B nodules do not occur alone. The main histological patterns of the lesions are similar in untreated mice and those on the long-term feeding with compounds. However, the cytology is modified by the compound used.

Type A nodules. Microscopic lesions are difficult to distinguish from the adjacent normal liver. They are composed of regular arrangements of closely packed cells and sinusoids compressing the surrounding liver (Fig. 3). The trabeculae are one cell and occasionally two cells thick. Normal mitoses are scattered throughout the lesion. Larger nodules, up to 1.5 to 2 cm diam. may consist entirely of this typical regular

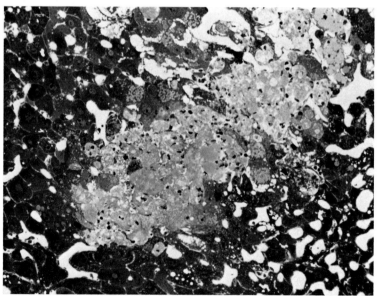

Fig. 6. A small infarct in a nodule induced by phenobarbitone 1000 ppm in the diet. Epoxy resin 1 μ section stained with toluidine blue $\times$ 160.

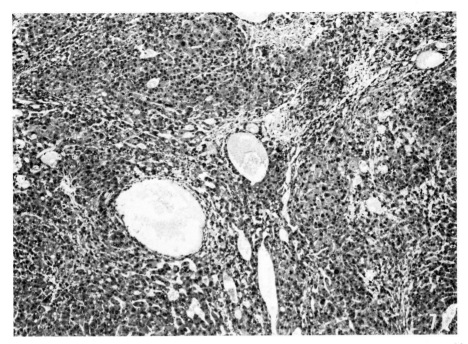

Fig. 7. Typical area from the centre of a large type A nodule illustrating the vascular spaces, atrophic trabeculae and small foci of scarring. Phenobarbitone 1000 ppm. H and E×144.

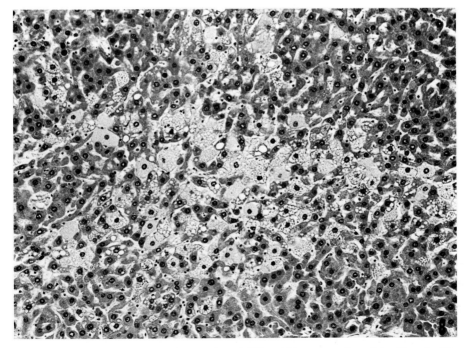

Fig. 8. A group of pale vacuolated parenchymal cells within a type A nodule. Phenobarbitone 1000 ppm. H and E×144.

pattern. The vessels of the portal tracts and central veins of the surrounding tissue becomes stretched around the rim of the expanding lesion (Figs. 3 and 4). Large vascular spaces and small areas of infarction occur in the centre of the larger lesions (Figs. 5 and 6). Areas of atrophic trabeculae, thin single cords expanded by each nucleus surrounded by wide sinusoids, and small foci of fibrosis and scarring are also seen (Fig. 7). Occasionally lesions contain necrotic haemorrhagic areas associated with cells of typical A morphology. Other variations found in these large nodules are small foci of basophilic cells, proliferating foci within a larger nodule, areas of fatty degeneration (Fig. 8), extensive vacuolation of the cells and hyaline droplet change. All these are associated with a basically regular parenchymal cell pattern in the nodules. The individual cell morphology of the nodules is dependent on the compound used. Lesions in control mice consist of small regular cells, uni- or binucleate (Figs. 4 and 9). The nuclei have few nucleoli and occasional inclusions (Fig. 10). A few large nuclei are found in most nodules from control mice over 0.5 cm diam. Larger eosinophilic cells with bizarre nuclei and inclusions are characteristic of compound induced nodules (Figs. 26, 28, 29, 30). These changes will be discussed later.

Type B nodules. Small foci occur within large type A nodules of irregular papillary structure. These are typical of type B lesions and range in size from a few mm to several cm in diam. The orderly trabecular pattern is lost, wide papillary forms with trabeculae 5 to 6 cells thick are common (Figs. 11, 12, 13 and 14). Haemorrhage and necrosis occur in the majority of these lesions. Areas of atrophy (Figs. 15 and 16) scarring, calcification and infarction are common. Other parenchymal cell patterns occur. Adenomatous forms are seen consisting of small regular cells arranged in glandular fashion and surrounded by connective tissue stroma (Fig. 17) and more

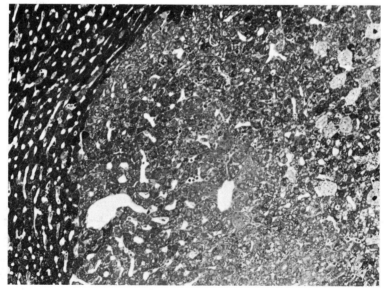

Fig. 9. Edge of type A nodule from a control mouse. Epoxy resin 1 μ section stained with toluidine blue. $\times 130$.

cystic lesion with large spaces surrounded by flattened parenchymal cells (Fig. 18). This latter lesion may arise from necrosis of the central portion of a papillary lesion and an intermediate phase is frequently seen affecting a proportion of the trabeculae (Fig. 19). As in the type A lesion fatty degeneration and vacuolation of the cells occur (Fig. 8). The mitotic rate is raised in these lesions, however, undifferentiated foci are rarely, if ever, seen. Similar to the A lesions, these B nodules compress the surrounding liver. Evidence of local invasion, especially vessel invasion, is difficult to find.

Cytological appearance of the nodules. The effect of individual compounds on the cytology of the liver cells in the nodules and the surrounding liver has been alluded to previously. DDT, dieldrin and phenobarbitone are inducers of mixed function oxidases and cause proliferation of the smooth endoplasmic reticulum (SER) of the hepatocytes which is most marked in the centrilobular zone. Chronic feeding of phenobarbitone produces a gradation of changes throughout the lobule with large eosinophilic centrilobular cells (Fig. 20). In epoxy resin embedded 1 μ sections they appear pale and empty and electron microscopy shows them to contain dilated SER. The nuclei are large and frequently of bizarre shapes (dumb-bell, infolded) and an occasional cell is multinucleate (Fig. 21). These are confined to the area adjacent to the central vein. Large nuclear inclusions are common consisting of fat and recognizable cytoplasmic organelles. The nucleoli are increased in number and the chromatin pattern variable. Cells around the portal tracts are smaller with more uniform nuclear morphology. Isolated necrotic cells with an appropriate macrophage reaction can be found in the affected zones, and a low grade mitotic response to this and perhaps the inducing drug occurs. In a few mice scattered small infarcts occur throughout the non-tumour bearing liver (Fig. 22).

The cytological changes seen in the nodules are similar to those described above occurring in the remaining liver. The cells from induced nodules are larger than those from untreated mice and many stain intensely eosinophilic (Figs. 23 and 24). Nuclei vary in size, many are four to five times normal size (Fig. 25) with multiple nucleoli (Fig. 26), inclusions (Figs. 27, 28 and 29) and infoldings (Fig. 30). Multinucleate cells characteristic of the centrilobular change (Fig. 21) are not found within the nodules. The nuclear abnormalities described occur in nodules from untreated mice (Fig. 10) but they are seen infrequently. Both type A and B test nodules contain these bizarre forms. The nuclear pleomorphism does not correlate well with the histological pattern. DDT and dieldrin both produce similar changes in mouse liver but the picture is less pronounced than with phenobarbitone (Figs. 28 and 30). Metastasising lesions in untreated animals may have uniform nuclear morphology (Fig. 13).

A preliminary EM study of the nodules induced in C3H mice by phenobarbitone has demonstrated several ultrastructural differences between the nodules in test and control animals. Material fixed by vascular perfusion *in vivo* and embedded in epoxy resin show a uniformity of organization throughout the nodules in both groups (Figs. 9 and 31). It is difficult to place these lesions in either A or B category. On the other hand, the cytological differences, especially those of nuclear size and morphology (Fig. 25), are striking in this well fixed material but as in the paraffin-embedded series, similar changes are found in the liver outside these nodules. Nucleoli through-

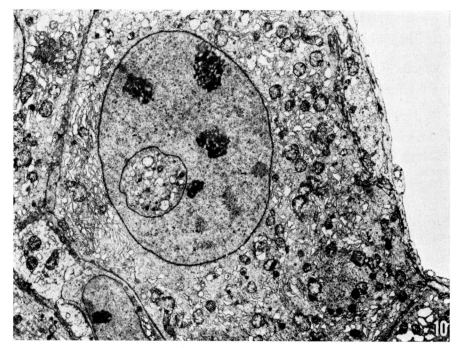

Fig. 10. Large nuclear inclusion found in a parenchymal cell nodule in a control mouse. EM × 4000.

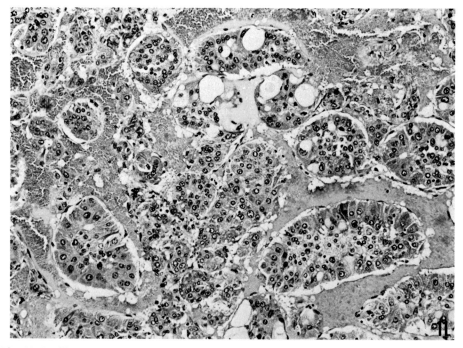

Fig. 11. Papillary area in a type B lesion induced by acetylaminofluorene 0·03% in diet. H and E × 144 (P. M. Newberne).

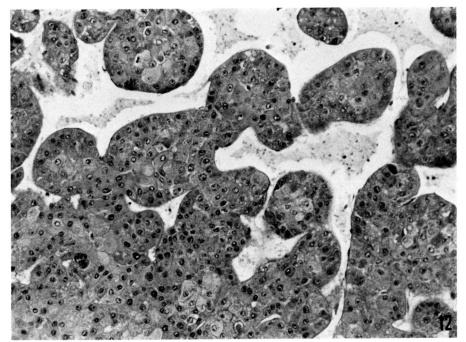

Fig. 12. Papillary area in a type B lesion induced by Scarlet Red 600 ppm in the diet. H and E × 184 (E. THORPE).

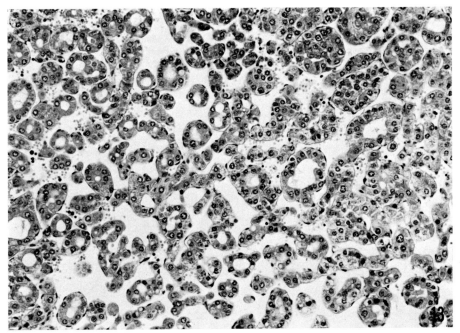

Fig. 13. Adenomatous area from a type B lesion in a control mouse. Note the regular cell morphology illustrated. H and E × 144.

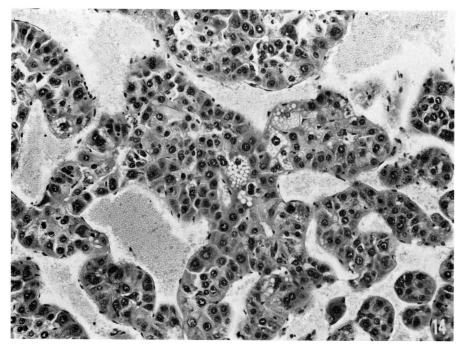

Fig. 14. Papillary area from a type B lesion induced by phenobarbitone. Note the foci of vacuolated cells and the range of nuclear size and morphology in the trabeculae. H and E × 144.

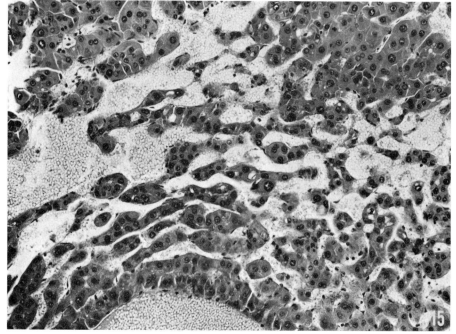

Fig. 15. Thinned atrophic trabeculae within a type B nodule. Phenobarbitone 1000 ppm in the diet. H and E × 144.

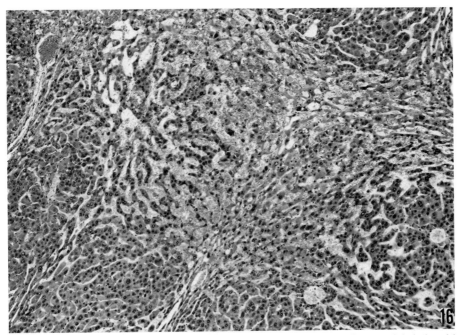

Fig. 16. Low power photomicrograph of a vascular area from the centre of a B nodule induced by phenobarbitone 1000 ppm in the diet. H and E×144.

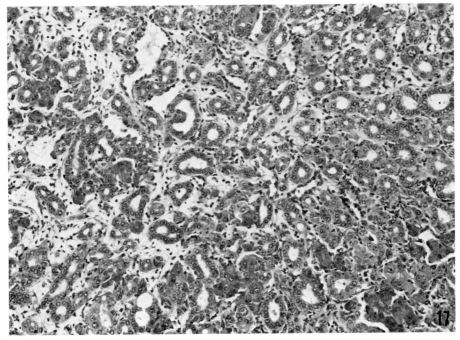

Fig. 17. Focus of typical adenomatous pattern within a parenchymal cell nodule induced by Scarlet Red. H and E×144 (E. Thorpe).

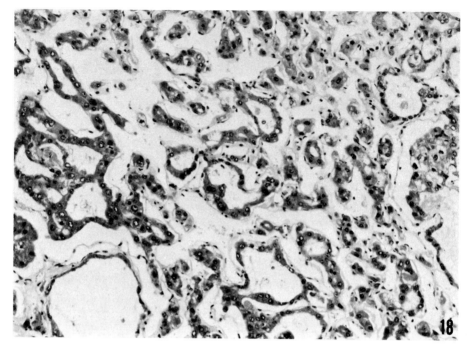

Fig. 18. Area of cystic change within a nodule induced by DDT. H and E×144 (L. TOMATIS).

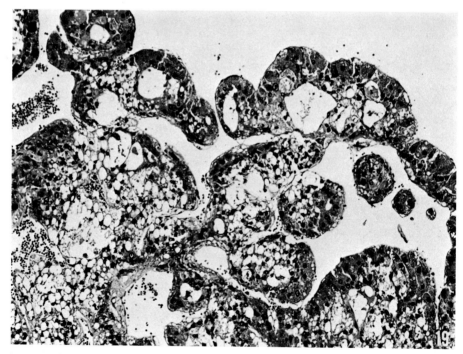

Fig. 19. Papillary area from a type B lesion induced by DDT. Note the cystic change and necrosis in the centre of the larger trabeculae. H and E×144 (E. THORPE).

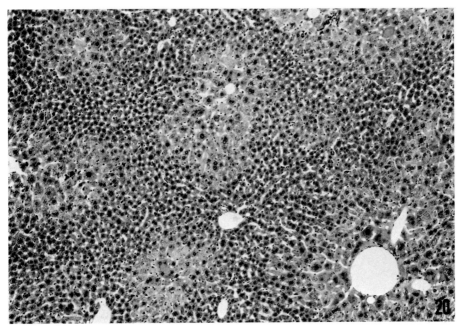

Fig. 20. Low power photomicrograph illustrating the cellular changes produced by phenobarbitone in the centrilobular areas outside the nodules. H and E × 56.

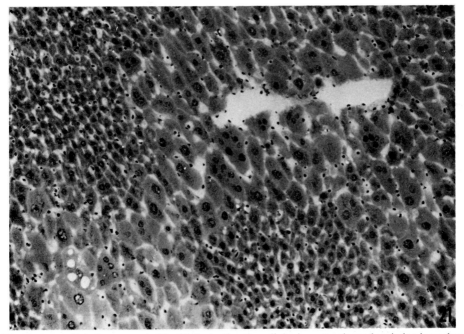

Fig. 21. A centrilobular zone as in Fig. 20 illustrating the cellular hypertrophy and variation in nuclear size induced by phenobarbitone. Note the occasional multinucleate cell immediately adjacent to the central vein. H and E × 160.

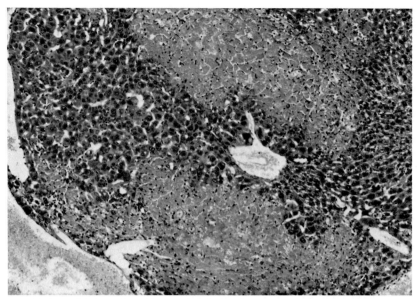

Fig. 22. Multiple small infarcts found in non-tumour bearing areas of liver. Phenobarbitone 1000 ppm in the diet. H and E × 80.

out the liver in the test groups are increased in number and abnormal in structure (Fig. 32). No abnormal mitosis was seen. The liver cell plates within the control and induced nodules are lined by normal endothelial cells and basement membrane (Fig. 33). Groups of active macrophages are plentiful in both test and control groups (Figs. 34 and 35). The significance of their presence and activity is under investigation. Occasional necrotic cells are seen in the tissue studied in the EM and small infarcts within the nodules identified. The cytoplasm of the hepatocytes in the test nodules consists largely of areas of smooth endoplasmic reticulum similar to the extensive proliferation found in the centrilobular hepatocytes described previously (Fig. 36). Smooth endoplasmic reticulum is sparse in hepatocytes of nodules from control mice (Figs. 37 and 38).

Lung metastases from these liver nodules are reported in controls and long-term feeding experiments with DDT, dieldrin and phenobarbitone. They range in size from several cm in diam. and are recognizable macroscopically (Fig. 39) to a few microns in diam. forming small tumour clumps of a few cells in the peripheral lung capillaries (Fig. 40). The morphology of these metastases is similar to that of the parent liver lesion (Fig. 41). Both control and compound-induced lesions are reported to metastasise but the incidence in all series is very low. In a study undertaken by WALKER, THORPE AND STEVENSON (1972) feeding dieldrin 0–10 ppm to CF1 mice for 132 weeks, 95 out of 585 control mice developed liver nodules. 11 of these were classified as type B lesions and 2 metastasised. 423 of 736 test mice in this experiment developed nodules, 203 of type B morphology and 9 of these metastasised. In a second similar study over 128 weeks feeding 0–20 ppm dieldrin, 6 B lesions metastasised from 244 test mice. No lesions from the control mice produced metastases. Long-term feeding

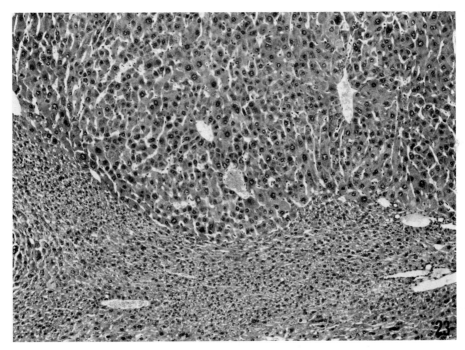

Fig. 23. The edge of a type A nodule induced by phenobarbitone 1000 ppm in the diet. The lesion is compressing the adjacent normal liver. There is no evidence of invasion. H and E×56.

of DDT, up to 250 ppm, to a total of 1000 mice produced 4 metastasising lesions, and none in the control series of 224 (TOMATIS *et al.*, 1972). Recently 1000 ppm phenobarbitone in the diet has been reported as giving metastasising B lesions in 8 of 30 CF1 mice (THORPE, unpublished observations). Also in an unpublished series, P. M. NEWBERNE (personal communication) has found that 0·03% acetylaminofluorene for 14 months induced 52% incidence of liver nodules (26/50) of which 8 metastasised. Histologically the liver nodules were similar to the type B lesions (Fig. 11).

Vascular lesions. Vascular nodules arising in mouse liver cover a wide range of morphological types. A brief selection will be discussed here. A vascular lesion occurring after DMN treatment is illustrated in Fig. 42. It consists of large vascular spaces surrounded by a normal single cell trabeculum and lined by normal vascular endothelium (Fig. 43). There is no increase in the mitotic rate. Areas of laminated thrombus within the vascular space and the surrounding active fibroblasts and macrophage response provide questionable evidence of malignancy of this type of lesion (Fig. 44).

Haemorrhagic lesions with many features in common with this have been reported in mice treated with urethane (KAWAMOTO *et al.*, 1961; TRAININ, 1963). The liver may be enlarged two to three times normal size by multiple blood-filled cysts, surrounded by normal or compressed liver parenchyma. Blood clot and thrombus occur and in some areas resemble cavernous haemangioma. Cellular proliferation, granulation tissue, at the edge of the cysts and associated with thrombus or clot have led to this

38

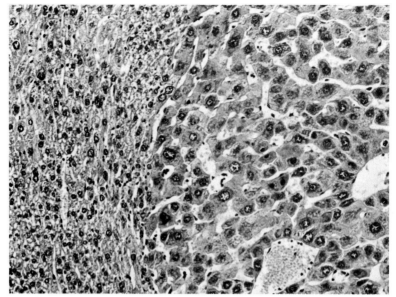

Fig. 24. High power photomicrograph of the edge of the lesion illustrated in Fig. 23. Note the increased size of the cells within the nodule, the presence of mitosis and the compressing edge. H and E×160.

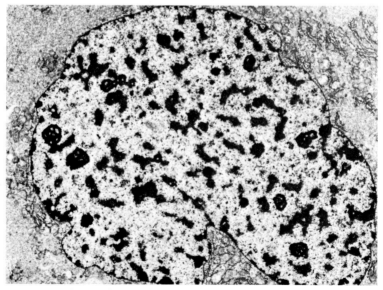

Fig. 25. A low power electronmicrograph of a bizarre nucleus within a type B nodule induced by phenobarbitone. ×3000.

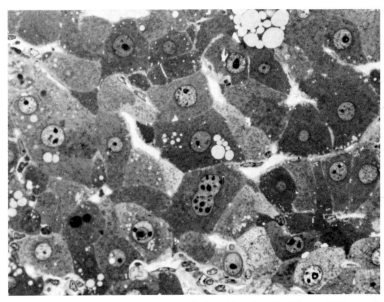

Fig. 26. Nuclear abnormalities found in nodules induced by phenobarbitone 1000 ppm in the diet. A large "dumb-bell" shaped nucleus with multiple nucleoli is illustrated. Epoxy resin 1 μ section stained with toluidine blue. $\times 400$.

lesion being considered neoplastic. Further support to this view is the transplantibility of the lesions demonstrated by TRAININ in C57 Black 6 mice and by DERINGER (1962) in HR-DE mice.

Other proliferative lesions of the endothelium of the liver sinusoids give the more characteristic appearance of haemangioendothelioma. Parenchymal cells surround dilated sinusoids, lined by plump active endothelial cells (Fig. 45). In the example illustrated, small foci of tumour were found scattered throughout the liver distant to the main mass, indicating local invasion. This lesion was induced by DMN. In C3H mice fed 25 ppm DMN in the diet undifferentiated vascular tumours occur in the liver (Fig. 46). These are frequently multifocal within the liver and are found in addition in other organs including lung, kidney and spleen. The lesions are composed of loose nests of intensely basophilic cells with pyknotic hyperchromatic nuclei between strands of parenchymal cells. Areas of necrosis, haemorrhage and cystic degeneration occur and the vascular cells invade the adjacent normal liver (Fig. 47). The morphology of the lesion in lung, kidney and spleen is similar to the liver. The lungs may contain multiple such lesions and in addition evidence of secondary spread from extrapulmonary sites (Fig. 48). Small plugs of tumour cells blocking the peribronchial and peripheral lung capillaries can be found. This highly malignant vascular lesion in multiple sites is best described as an angiosarcoma.

Tumours arising from the bile duct. The characteristic tumour consisting of acinar structures and associated fibroblastic response is not found in mice. Cholangiomas are reported in C3H/AvyfB mice and their hybrids with BALB-C (VLAHAKIS AND HESTON, 1971) and in C3H mice (REUBER, 1967). The authors indicate that these

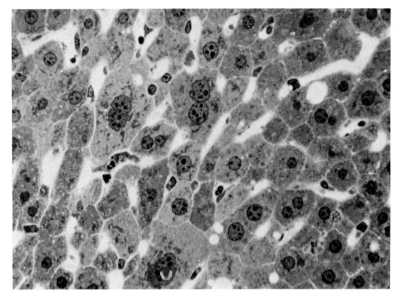

Fig. 27. Multiple nucleoli and nuclear inclusions seen within a nodule induced by phenobarbitone. Epoxy resin 1 μ section stained with H and E $\times$ 460.

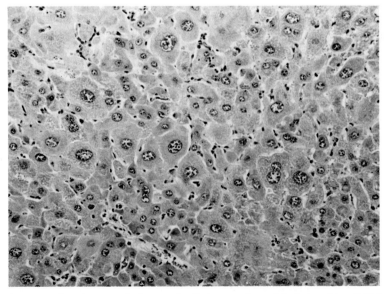

Fig. 28. The range of nuclear morphology and cell size seen in nodule induced by dieldrin 10 ppm in the diet. Nuclei of bizarre shape and size containing inclusions are illustrated. H and E $\times$ 132 (E. THORPE).

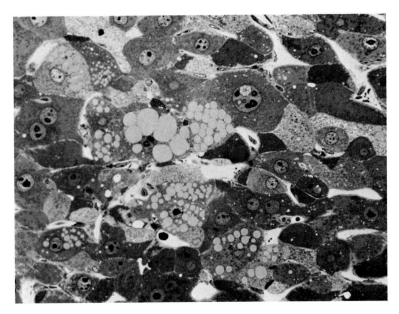

Fig. 29. Part of the nodule illustrated in Fig. 26. A small focus of cells containing fat both in the cytoplasm and nuclei is illustrated. Epoxy resin 1 μ section stained with toluidine blue. ×320.

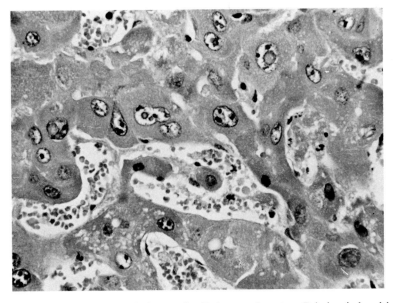

Fig. 30. The range of nuclear morphology and cell size seen in a type B lesion induced by DDT. Several nuclei contain inclusions and multiple nucleoli. H and E×330 (E. Thorpe).

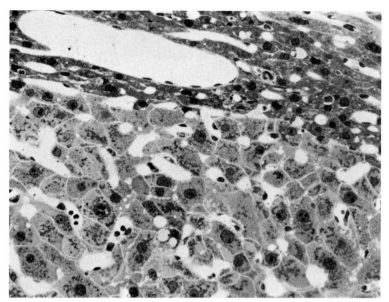

Fig. 31. Edge of nodule induced by phenobarbitone 1000 ppm in the diet. Epoxy resin 1 μ section stained with H and E $\times$ 330.

lesions may arise in "hepatomas" and consist of sheets of uniform cells with large dark nuclei, at first lining cystic spaces and later forming solid tumours (Fig. 49). The well differentiated varieties are described forming duct-like structures. Mitotic activity is high and areas of cystic change, haemorrhage and necrosis occur. The possibility that these lesions are mesenchymal in origin has been suggested as the cells lack typical epithelial characteristics and the lesion does not resemble the cholangiocarcinomas of other species. Of 296 C3H/AvyfB mice 23 had cholangiomas at autopsy. One of these lesions was transplanted into 3 females of the same strain; the same tumour produced a lung metastasis.

Reticuloendothelial tumours. Spontaneous and compound induced lesions have been reported (DUNN, 1954). These are extrahepatic neoplasms which form the commonest secondary tumour found in mouse liver. The proliferating reticuloendothelial cells form solid masses around the portal tracts and central veins. (Fig. 50) Occasionally a diffuse infiltration of the sinusoids occurs. This diffuse pattern is also found within proliferative parenchymal lesions in the liver (Fig. 51).

DISCUSSION

The main problem that arises from the study of the nodular lesions in the mouse liver is making an assessment of their biological behaviour. It is obviously important to determine which of the lesions are carcinoma and to recognize the characteristics of the lesion which enables this diagnosis to be made. In the recommendations of the IARC Working Conference on Liver Cancer it was suggested that the assessment of

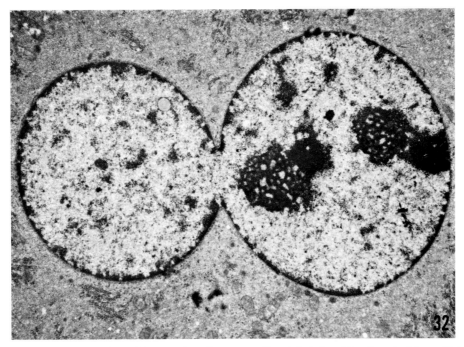

Fig. 32. "Dumb-bell" shaped large nucleus from a type B nodule induced by phenobarbitone. Note the abnormal nucleoli. EM × 6920.

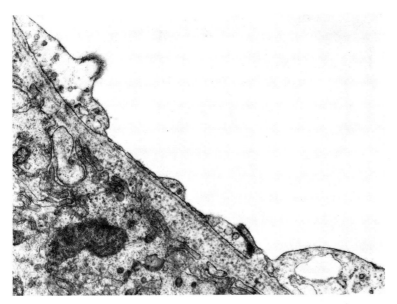

Fig. 33. The endothelial lining of the sinusoid within a nodule from a control mouse. Note the presence of basement membrane. EM × 6000.

44

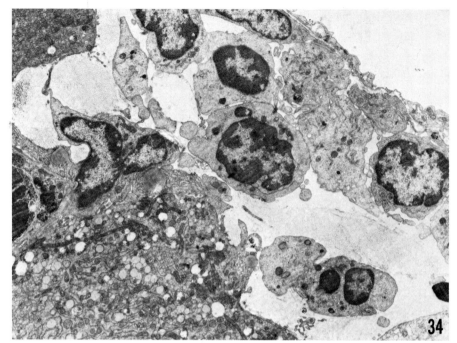

Fig. 34. A group of macrophages and mononuclear cells lying between the parenchymal cells and the endothelial lining of the sinusoids. A type B nodule induced by phenobarbitone. EM × 4000.

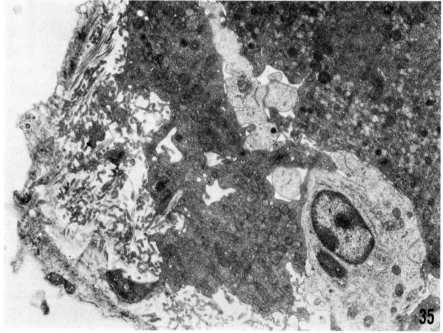

Fig. 35. A macrophage with cytoplasmic extensions between two adjacent parenchymal cells. A type B lesion induced by phenobarbitone. EM × 6400.

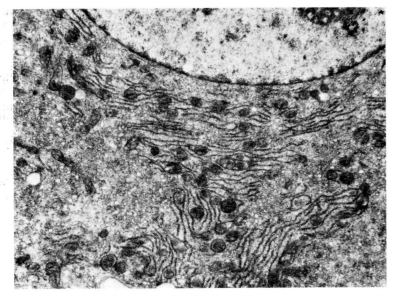

Fig. 36. Electronmicrograph of a typical parenchymal cell from a type A nodule induced by pheno-barbitone. Note the large amount of smooth endoplasmic reticulum within the cell. EM × 8000.

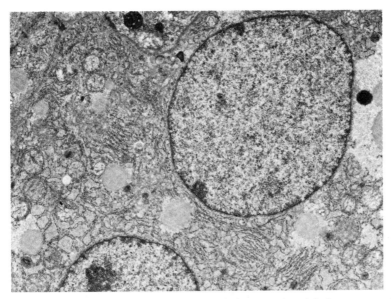

Fig. 37. Electronmicrograph of a typical parenchymal cell in a type A nodule from a control mouse. Note the normal nuclear morphology and the stacks of rough endoplasmic reticulum in the cyto-plasm. There is little smooth endoplasmic reticulum in these cells. EM × 5100.

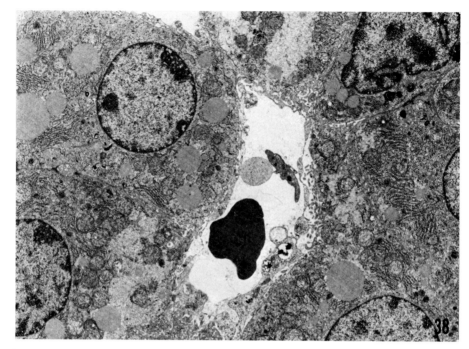

Fig. 38. Low power electronmicrograph of nodule in a control mouse. EM × 3200.

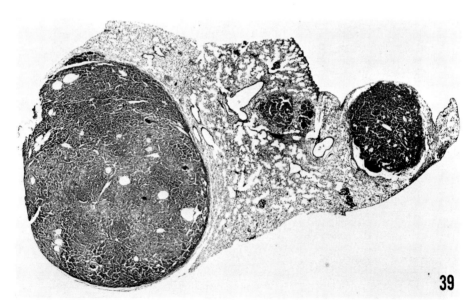

Fig. 39. Multiple large metastases from a type B liver lesion induced by dieldrin 2·6 ppm in the diet. H and E × 16 (E. THORPE).

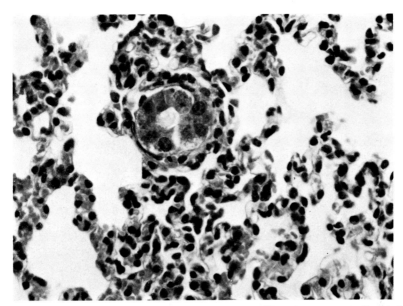

Fig. 40. Small tumour embolus blocking a peripheral lung capillary from a type B liver lesion in a control mouse. H and E × 460 (E. Thorpe).

the carcinogenicity of a lesion should be based upon its biological behaviour; that is the presence of invasion or metastases. However, in all published series and from our experience with phenobarbitone, the incidence of metastases is very low. Even in the reports (Walker et al., 1971) where the lungs were step serial sectioned metastases were only found in 2·1% of mice with nodules. In our own series we have so far failed to find any metastasis or evidence of local invasion. From literature surveys this would appear to be a common finding. Therefore, except in those cases where such biological behaviour can be demonstrated in a high incidence, the definitive diagnosis of carcinoma cannot be made.

In the earlier part of this paper we have attempted to sub-divide the parenchymal cell lesions using the criteria of Walker et al. (1971). This classification was initially used as a convenient but arbitrary division. Walker et al., also found that the metastases occurred in those animals with the type B lesions. This classification was primarily based upon the structure of the nodules and its associated vascular bed and secondarily upon the cytology. At the extreme ends of the spectrum we find it reasonably easy to make the distinction between the types of lesion. However, there appears to be a continuous spectrum of change without a sharp separation of types. On our large area plastic embedded material the subdivision of types becomes even less certain.

The cytological characteristics of the lesions have been used as diagnostic criteria of malignancy. In the large nodules arising in controls there is some variation in both cell size and staining characteristics of the cytoplasm, as well as increased variation in nuclear size. It is worth noting that in non-tumour bearing untreated mice, 18–24 months old, there is considerable variation in nuclear morphology. Multinucleate cells are also present and the nuclei contain cytoplasmic inclusions.

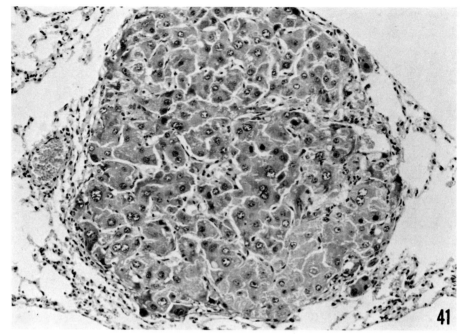

Fig. 41. Lung metastasis from a type B liver lesion induced by dieldrin 10 ppm in the diet. The morphology of the metastasis is similar to that of the primary liver lesion H and E × 144 (E. THORPE).

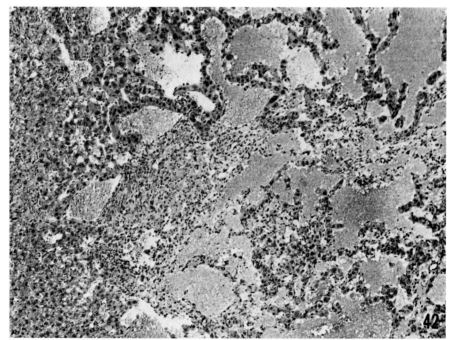

Fig. 42. Liver nodule containing large vascular spaces between strands of parenchymal cells. This lesion was induced by dimethylnitrosamine. H and E × 72 (L. DEN ENGELSE et al.).

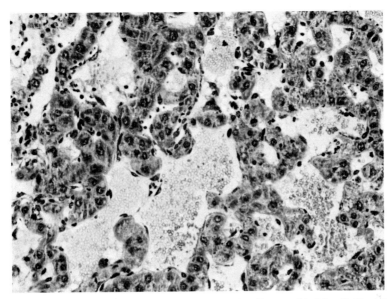

Fig. 43. Higher power photomicrograph of the vascular lesion illustrated in Fig. 42. Note the regular single cell strands of parenchymal cells. The vascular spaces are lined by normal endothelium. H and E × 200 (L. DEN ENGELSE et al.).

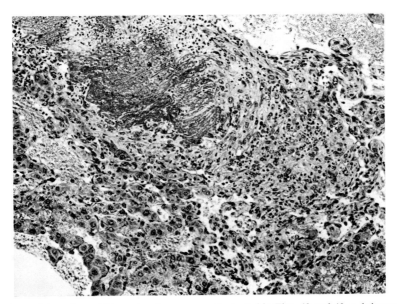

Fig. 44. Area of thrombus within a vascular space as illustrated in Figs. 42 and 43 and the associated cellular area of typical granulation tissue. H and E × 130 (L. DEN ENGELSE et al.).

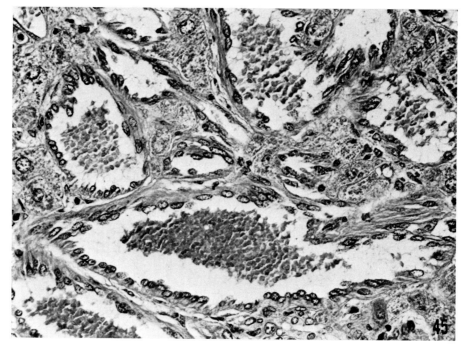

Fig. 45. Photomicrograph of a haemangioendothelioma induced by dimethylnitrosamine showing flattened endothelial cells lining the vascular spaces (L. DEN ENGELSE *et al.*).

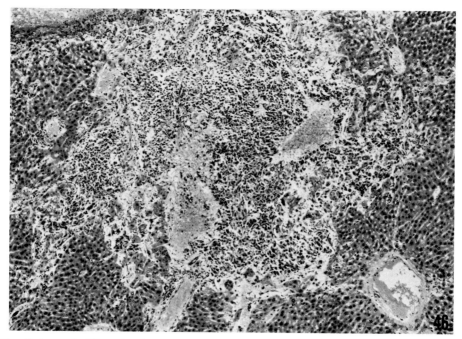

Fig. 46. A poorly differentiated vascular hepatic neoplasm induced by dimethylnitrosamine to show the local invasion of tumour and areas of haemorrhage and necrosis within it. H and E × 56.

In considering the cytology of the compound-induced lesions, especially where the compound is fed continuously, one must consider the effect of the compound upon the cytology, both within or without the nodules. In the nodular lesions induced by the pesticides DDT and dieldrin or by phenobarbitone there is considerable pleomorphism of both cytoplasmic or nuclear morphology (Figs. 26, 28, 29 and 30). The cytoplasm is more eosinophilic and in the case of phenobarbitone contains large areas of SER (Fig. 36). This gives an indication that the cells are able to respond to the inducing properties of phenobarbitone. There is some increased variation in mitochondrial morphology but this does not appear to be very marked. The nuclei show the greatest change with considerable variation in size and form often with multiple inclusions of fat and cytoplasm (Figs. 25, 29 and 32). These changes cannot be considered to be an indication of the neoplastic behaviour of the nodule as in the case of phenobarbitone all of these changes can be demonstrated in the non-nodular parts of the liver. That the nodules are proliferative is not doubted as the normal architecture is distorted and multiple mitotic figures are present in all lesions we have examined.

The study of neoplastic lesions in rodents is important for two reasons. Firstly to further the understanding of the pathogenesis of neoplasia and secondly as part of toxicological evaluation of new compounds. In both cases the extrapolation of the animal data to man must be based upon an evaluation of the information available. Therefore it is essential to attempt to get an accurate diagnosis of the proliferative lesions in the rat and mouse liver. The morphology and biological behaviour of these lesions in the rat has been described by many investigators. There is convincing evidence of a correlation between the structure of the primary lesion and its ability to invade and metastasize in the host. Also the incidence of metastases is high. In our experience with aflatoxin 75 % of rats with such pleomorphic lesions have demonstrable invasion and metastases. Therefore a diagnosis of hepatocellular carcinoma on the morphology of the primary liver lesion is justified.

In the mouse the situation is confused. There are only a few descriptions in the literature of the morphology of the lesions. There is even less published evidence of their biological behaviour in the host making any correlation between the morphology of the primary lesion and behaviour in the host unwise if not impossible. The presence of a 5% incidence of metastases from a defined lesion is insufficient evidence of the malignant nature of the remaining 95%. It can only arouse suspicion as to their nature.

Classification of focal proliferative liver lesions in the mouse into morphological types A and B provides a useful working scheme. Type A lesions have not been associated with invasion or metastases. Type B lesions have been associated with metastases in a few cases. Two explanations are possible for this apparent discrepancy between structure of the primary lesion and the presence of metastases as reported in the literature. First the lesions may be fundamentally different from those of similar morphology in the rat and hence do not represent malignant neoplasia in the mouse. Second a correct assessment of the lesions may not be possible because of insufficient sampling of organs and poor preparative technique. Both opinions must be considered

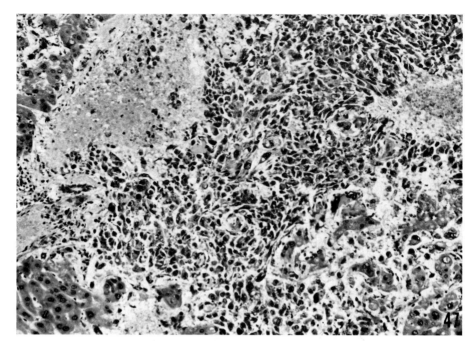

Fig. 47. A higher power photomicrograph of the lesion illustrated in Fig. 46. Note the bizarre irregular spindle-shaped cells invading between islands of parenchymal cells. H and E × 144.

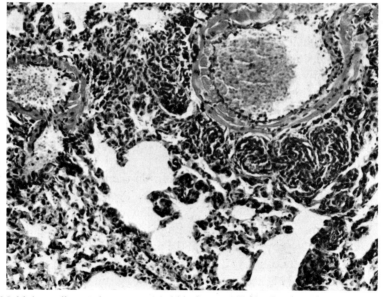

Fig. 48. Multiple small secondary tumours within lung capillaries from a primary extra-pulmonary vascular lesion. Dimethylnitrosamine 25 ppm in the diet. H and E × 160.

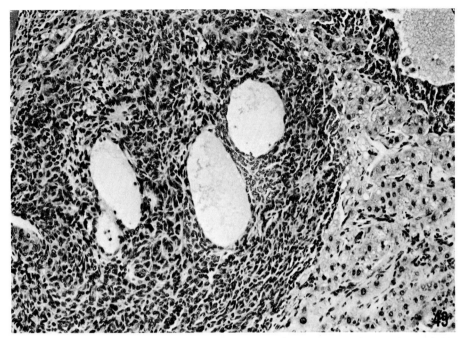

Fig. 49. The edge of a "cholangioma" with a few small cystic spaces and areas of an acinar formation. H and E × 144.

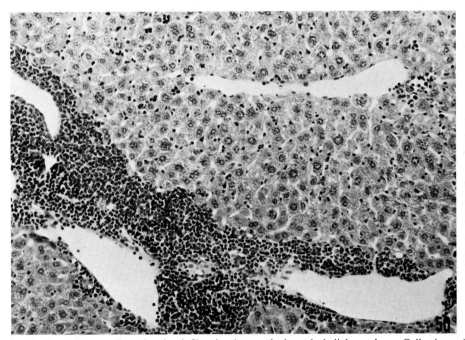

Fig. 50. Control mouse liver showing infiltration by a reticulo-endothelial neoplasm. Collections of basophilic cells occur around the portal tracts and central veins. H and E × 144.

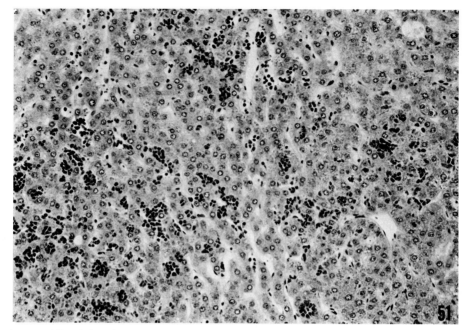

Fig. 51. Diffuse infiltration of a type A nodule of the control mouse in Fig. 50 by a reticulo-endo-thelial tumour. H and E × 144.

until further data are available. A diagnosis of hepatocellular carcinoma for B lesions in mice is an opinion based upon experience in other species. However, we consider it important that this opinion is based upon evidence derived from the mouse which at present is not available. When available, these data will provide a factual basis for the diagnosis.

The factors which influence the development of these lesions are little understood and will also be discussed by Dr. GRASSO and Dr. GELLATLY. However, two factors have arisen from this study. Firstly we have found possible virus-like particles (Fig. 52) in both control and induced lesions. Whether this is passenger virus or has a role in the induction of the lesion is not known. The other possible major factor is that the compounds themselves are both inducers of mixed function oxidases and in high doses hepatotoxic. In the course of the feeding experiments, parenchymal cell death occurs. In the older animals areas of infarction are found within and without the nodules. Loss of parenchymal cells in the non-nodular part of the liver would lead to hyperplasia. It is not known whether infarction within nodules would also stimulate a mitotic response within the nodule. The nodules induced by phenobarbitone are able to respond to the compound in that they have an increased amount of SER (Fig. 36). There is no information on whether the SER is functional in its ability to metabolise the inducing compound.

Vascular neoplasia presents less of a problem. In many studies, haemangioendotheliomas have been reported (ANDERVONT AND GRADY, 1942; SALAMAN AND ROE, 1953; ROE, 1954; HESTON et al., 1960; KAWAMOTO et al., 1961; TRAININ, 1963; SEVERI

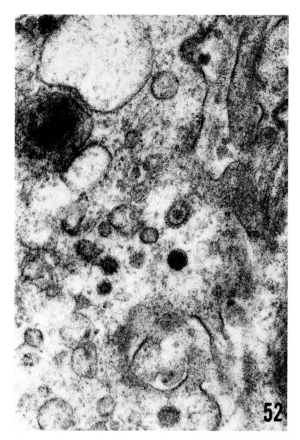

Fig. 52. High power electronmicrograph of the cytoplasm of a parenchymal cell in a control nodule illustrating possible virus particles within these cells. EM × 52 500.

AND BIANCIFIORI, 1968; TAKAYAMA AND OOTA, 1965) but it would appear that two distinct forms are seen. The first is the lesion induced by the nitrosamines (TAKAYAMA AND OOTA, 1965), and not reported in controls, and discussed by Dr. TAKAYAMA (Chapter 4) at this meeting. We have also induced this lesion by feeding 25 ppm DMN to male C3H mice. The neoplasm appears as an anaplastic mesenchymal lesion invading the surrounding tissue (Figs. 46 and 47) and metastasises to the lung (Fig. 48). This lesion is also found in the kidney, spleen and lungs which might suggest a multicentric origin. The more cellular portions of this neoplasm resemble the rat renal angiosarcoma induced by DMN (HARD AND BUTLER, 1970). Dr. TAKAYAMA (Chapter 4) has reported that this neoplasm is derived from the sinusoid lining cells but a detailed study of the fully developed sarcoma remains to be done.

The second form of vascular neoplasm is a less well defined entity. This lesion consists of widely dilated vascular spaces lined by apparently normal endothelium (Figs. 42 and 43) and is seen in both control and treated mice. It is uncertain at present how true vascular neoplasia can be distinguished from a reactive telangectasis. The lesions vary from unilocular blood-filled spaces seen in old control mice to complex lesions. These lesions have been considered to resemble cavernous haemangioma (ROE, 1954) while BERENBLUM AND HARAN (1965) and TANNENBAUM AND SILVERSTONE (1958) considered the lesion to be reactive. In some cases invasion has been described (ANDERVONT AND GRADY, 1942) and also successful transplantation (TRAININ, 1963). At present no further conclusions can be drawn from the published work on how to differentiate the reactive from the neoplastic lesions.

In summary the main point to be made from study of the morphology of mouse hepatic neoplasia is that, within the host animal following treatment with some compounds, there does not appear to be a good correlation between morphological appearance of the lesion and its biological behaviour. In considering the parenchymal cell lesions, if the degree of organizational disturbance and cellular pleomorphism reflected the biological behaviour of the lesion within the animal, one might expect those experiments which have been reported in which there is a detailed description of the histology that an increasing incidence of pleomorphic lesions would parallel an increased incidence in obvious metastasis. From the literature this is not apparent.

REFERENCES

ANDERVONT, H. B., AND GRADY, H. G., AND EDWARDS, J. E. (1942). Induction of hepatic lesions, hepatomas, pulmonary tumours and haemangioendotheliomas in mice with *o*-aminoazotoluene. *J. Natl. Cancer Inst.*, 3: 131.

ANDERVONT, H. B., AND DUNN, T. B. (1952) Transplantation of spontaneous and induced hepatomas in inbred mice. *J. Natl. Cancer Inst.*, 13: 455.

BERENBLUM, I., AND HARAN, N. (1955) The initiating action of ethyl carbamate (urethane) on mouse skin. *Brit. J. Cancer*, 9: 453.

CLAPP, N. K., AND CRAIG, A. W. (1967) Carcinogenic effects of diethylnitrosamine in RF mice. *J. Natl. Cancer Inst.*, 39: 903.

DERINGER, M. K. (1962) Response of strain HR-DE mice to painting with urethan. *J. Natl. Cancer Inst.*, 39: 903.

DERINGER, M. K. (1962) Response of strain HR-DE mice to painting with urethan. *J. Natl. Cancer Inst.*, 29: 1107.

DUNN, T. B. (1954) Normal and pathologic anatomy of the reticular tissue in laboratory mice, with a classification and discussion of neoplasms. *J. Natl. Cancer Inst.*, 14: 1281.

EDWARDS, J. E., AND DALTON, A. J. (1942). Induction of cirrhosis of the liver and of hepatomas in mice with carbon telrachloride. *J. Natl. Cancer Inst.*, 3: 19.

HARD, G. C., AND BUTLER, W. H. (1970) Cellular analysis of renal neoplasia: Induction of renal tumours in dietary conditioned rats by dimethylnitrosamine with a reappraisal of morphological characteristics. *Cancer Res.*, 30: 2796.

HESTON, W. E., VLAHAKIS, G., AND DERINGER, M. K. (1960) High incidence of spontaneous hepatomas and the increase of this incidence with urethan in C3H, C3Hf, and C3He male mice. *J. Natl. Cancer Inst.*, 24: 425.

KAWAMOTO, S., KIRSCHBAUM, A., IBANEZ, M. L., TRENTIN, J. J., AND TAYLOR, H. G. (1961) Influence of urethan on the development of spontaneous leukemia and on the induction of hemangiomas in the AKR and C58 strains of mice. *Cancer Res.*, 21/1: 71.

PERAINO, C., FRAY, R. J. M., AND STAFFELDT, E., (1973) Brief communication: Enhancement of spontaneous hepatic tumorigenesis in C3H mice by dietary phenobarbital. *J. Natl. Cancer Inst.*, 51: 1349.

REUBER, M. D. (1967) Poorly differentialed cholangiocarcinomas occurring "spontaneously" in C3H and C3Hxy hybrid mice. *J. Natl. Cancer Inst.*, 38: 901.

ROE, F. J. C. (1954). Liver changes in urethane-treated mice appearing after a long latent interval. *32nd Annual Report of the British Empire Cancer Campaign*, p. 170.

SALAMAN, M. H., AND ROE, F. J. C. (1953) Incomplete carcinogens: Ethylcarbamate (urethane) as an initiator of skin tumour formation in the mouse. *Brit. J. Cancer*, 7: 472.

SEVERI, L., AND BIANCIFIORI, C. (1968) Hepatic carcinogenesis in CBA/Cb/Se mice and Cb/Se rats by isonicotinic acid hydrazide and hydrazine sulfate. *J. Natl. Cancer Inst.*, 41: 331.

TAKAYAMA, S., AND OOTA, K. (1965) Induction of malignant tumours in various strains of mice by oral administration of N-nitrosodimethylamine and N-nitrosodiethylamine. *Gann (Jap. J. Cancer Res.)*, 56: 189.

TAKAYAMA, S., AND INUI, N. (1967) Induction of malignant tumours in mice fed (N,N-fluoren-2,7-ylene)bis acetylamine 27 FAA. *Gann. (Jap. J. Cancer Res.)*, 58: 193.

TANNENBAUM, A., AND SILVERSTONE, H. (1958) Urethan (ethyl carbamate) as a multipotential carcinogen. *Cancer Res.*, 18: 1225.

THORPE, E., AND WALKER, A. I. T. (1973) The toxicology of dieldrin (HEOD), II. Comparative long-term oral toxicity studies in mice with dieldrin, DDT, phenobarbitone, β-BHC and γ-BHC. *Food, Cosmet. Toxicol.*, 11: 433.

TOMATIS, L., TURUSOV, V., DAY, N., AND CHARLES, R. T. (1972) The effect of long-term exposure to DDT on CF-1 mice. *Int. J. Cancer*, 10: 489.

TRAININ, N. (1963) Neoplastic nature of liver "Blood Cysts" induced by urethan in mice. *J. Natl. Cancer Inst.*, 31/6: 1489.

VLAHAKIS, G., AND HESTON, W. E. (1971) Spontaneous cholangiomas in strain C3H-AvyfB mice and in their hybrids. *J. Natl. Cancer Inst.*, 46: 677.

WALKER, A. I. T., THORPE, E., AND STEVENSON, D. E. (1973) The toxicology of dieldrin (HEOD), I. Long-term oral toxicity studies in mice. *Food, Cosmet. Toxicol.*, 11: 415.

DISCUSSION

P. M. NEWBERNE. The most important thing which we must talk about now are those lesions in which we do not have metastases. We are never going to have metastases in 100% of cases, therefore, what are the criteria for deciding which of the 95% of the non-metastasizing lesions are malignant neoplasia. We will have to decide on how to make this diagnosis, otherwise we will never be able to deal with those regulatory authorities who have to make decisions on the use of compounds and drugs. It is the purpose of this meeting to come to grips with this problem and try and define those lesions which are malignant but which we cannot clearly say are such on the basis of the fact of the presence of metastases. Dr. TAKAYAMA (Appendix I) has shown that if you send a series of slides to different pathologists you get very different opinions. This is a common observation.

REUBER. Very few studies have been done to investigate the true incidence of metastases and further no good studies have been done to demonstrate the presence of invasion. One section of a liver is not adequate. If animals are killed at the stage at which I consider that a nodule is becoming malignant, that is part of a nodule contains malignant cells and it is easy to miss the presence of malignant cells, the possibility of metastases at that stage is slight. However, I feel confident that if the mice were withdrawn from the chemical and allowed to live for two more years, that is a total of four years, we would have metastases in all the animals and they would be killed by the carcinoma. I consider that we have to make the diagnosis of neoplasia on the histological and cytological characteristics of the lesions and that this is adequate.

BUTLER. It is often suggested that if one waits long enough the animals will produce metastases. This is an impossible situation. If a mouse lived for twenty years you may be right, but mice do not live for that length of time. Therefore you have to consider the incidence of a lesion within a normal expected life span of the animal. In most published work the mice have not been deliberately killed early. Most investigators have waited until either the animals died or were moribund. It is reasonable to suggest that, if there is an increasing incidence of the lesion in question but the life span is not modified, then the lesion is not carcinoma. I agree that most studies have not been thorough in the search for metastases. In contrast to the mouse, in the rat there is little difficulty in finding metastases. If the 2–4% incidence is correct in the mouse, an explanation is required of the interpretation of carcinoma in this lesion. The problem is, is there a correlation between the morphology of the lesion in the mouse and its behaviour? I would suggest that there is not.

GELLATLY. In C57 black mice, we find solitary type B nodules without A nodules in the same liver. Further in our control series, we have found 1550 nodules of which 109 were classified as B. Nine of these had readily demonstrable metastases and, on step serial sections of 6 others, metastases were demonstrated in 3. A colleague examined a further 10 and failed to find metastases. In a study using butter yellow, 48% of mice survived to the end of the study at 80 weeks, and the incidence of metastases was similar to that in the controls, despite the fact that 79% of the mice had multiple nodules which could be classified as type B. When the study was extended from 80 to 100 weeks, there was no increase in the type B lesions or in the incidence of metastases.

THORPE. From our experience in mice treated with phenobarbitone, metastases occur late. It would therefore appear essential that the mice live 70 and 80 weeks in order to demonstrate metastases.

HOLLANDER. Do you include as metastases cells lying within a vessel? I do not consider them metastases. They are tumour emboli. We know from man that after operation or palpation of tumour we get cells spread throughout the body. If these emboli cannot be demonstrated to be growing, I would be against them being tabulated as metastases.

ROE. It is necessary to distinguish between cells which have just survived and those which multiply. Even though some may still be within vessels, they are obviously multiplying. I agree that they are emboli, but I would bracket them with metastases. We are discussing whether tumour emboli, with or without growth, is an absolute criterion for the diagnosis of malignancy. Nobody really disagrees that, if there is blood vessel invasion and spread, the lesion is malignant. I would agree that a distinction should be made between emboli and metastases, but I am sure that we would also agree that both are evidence of malignant neoplasia.

LEONARD. Do you therefore consider that those lesions which have the same morphology as metastasising lesions, but where metastases have not been demonstrated are malignant?

ROE. I would say I do not know.

BUTLER. This is obviously the main problem; in the mouse there is a low reported incidence of metastases. Do you consider that if one finds a type of lesion from 95% of which it is not possible to demonstrate metastases and 5% which metastasizes, you can extrapolate from the 5% to the 95%? I would consider that this is not reasonable. One has to attempt to recognise the morphological features associated with metastases. To me it is an unjustified extrapolation from a small number to a large number. Lesions should be described, but you must make clear that the extrapolation from the small group to the large group is an opinion.

THORPE. We must be most careful in this context. In a mouse you are not trying to make a prognosis based on the histology. In man the experience is such enabling one to make a prediction. But in our situation, we make a morphological classification and at this stage it would be a little rash to say that this should be regarded fundamentally as carcinoma. This concept was spelt out in the IARC Working Conference on Liver Cancer. These lesions look like carcinoma but there is a lack of information that they behave the same way as they do in the rat or other species.

REUBER. Without doubt, you can diagnose carcinoma on morphological features. In human pathology we do not require the presence of metastases in order to diagnose malignancy.

LAQUEUR. In man it is quite correct that we make the diagnosis upon the histological criteria with a high degree of accuracy. On histological grounds alone, I would classify the simple type A lesion described here as adenomas and the B lesion as hepatocarcinomas. However, when in doubt we should err on the conservative side.

GRASSO. The distinction between tumours that arise from haemangioendothelial tissue, bile-duct epithelium or from hepatic parenchymal cells does not seem to present a major problem. Further, there is little controversy on the nature of tumours of haemangioendothelial and bile-duct origin.

I think there is sufficient evidence from published work to enable a distinction to be made between well differentiated adenocarcinoma and benign nodular lesions. However, the further distinction of benign lesions into adenomas and hyperplastic lesions is extremely difficult. One is tempted to ask whether this distinction is worth making. Indeed, if one had in mind only the health of the mouse, such an effort would hardly be worth making unless there were clear indications that these nodules were associated with some non-neoplastic pathological process which threatens the survival of the animal. The evidence from many workers tends to show that there is no such association.

However, a distinction between hepatic adenomas and hyperplastic nodules becomes an urgent necessity in view of the tendency of many experimentalists to consider the induction of these hepatic nodular lesions as evidence of a carcinogenic response. There is evidence derived from both experimental work and observation of naturally occurring lesions, which suggests that the neoplastic process is a continuum from hyperplasia to frank malignancy. There is nevertheless equally good evidence that this progression is not obligatory, and the process may stop at any of the stages preceding frank malignancy and may even regress at some of the early stages [Shabad (1973) *J. Natl. Cancer Inst.*, 50: 1421]. There is no reason to suspect that this latter state of affairs may not be true for the mouse hepatic lesion, so that it is possible to envisage a situation where hyperplastic nodules are induced but do not progress further.

On what basis could a distinction be made between nodular hyperplasia and hepatic adenoma? Obviously no absolute criteria can be presented. In their absence one is justified in paying regard to the feeling of those pathologists who have devoted a considerable time and effort to the study of the problem. As far as could be judged from the limited papers available, nodules less than 5 mm at necropsy have not been considered as evidence of carcinogenic activity by ANDERVONT AND DUNN (1950, *J. Natl. Cancer Inst.*, 13: 455). Although these authors did not explicitly consider such nodules as hyperplasia it is reasonable to assume that this is what they meant because, in their studies, benign and malignant tumours are considered as one entity—neoplastic lesions. Later authors were more explicit [ESSNER (1967) *Cancer Res.*, 27: 2137; CONFER AND STENGER (1966) *Cancer Res.*, 26: 384; REUBER (1971) *Brit. J. Cancer*, 25: 538] and considered lesions 5 mm or less as hyperplastic. If one accepts this, then perhaps one could classify larger lesions which resemble fairly closely the architecture of hepatic parenchymal cords and do not display any of the characteristics of malignancy, as benign lesions—true hepatomas. There is, however, one other situation to be taken into account. If these large lesions possess a recognisable lobular architecture, however distorted, then perhaps one could follow LEMON's (1967, in *Pathology of Laboratory Rats and Mice*, ed. E. COTCHIN AND F. J. C. ROE, Blackwell, Oxford) advice and call these lesions nodular hyperplasia despite their size. Equally, lesions smaller than 5 mm should be classed as carcinomas if they show a true adenoid and papilliform architecture.

HOLLANDER. In the early 1960s I did a study of the effect of chronic irritation in carcinogenesis in the mouse. The animals survived for their normal life span, and in a series of 600 I found 30 with lesions which at that time I classifided as hepatomas. Four had gross pulmonary metastases. Recently I went through the cases without knowing which had metastasised in order to try to predict which had metastasised. This I could not do. My opinion is that you cannot make the diagnosis of malignancy only on morphology. It is necessary to take into account the biological behaviour. I tend to call all these tumours low grade malignancy. We know that well differentiated low grade tumours, such as endocrine tumours in man, seldom metastasise, but there appears to be a progression from hyperplasia to malignant neoplasia. Therefore for practical purposes I put them in the classification of malignant tumours.

ROE. I disagree with the concept of the necessity of erring in experimental work. It is not necessary. When one is looking for facts, we do not have to err. You can say you don't know. On the problem of the types of lesion, the A and B classification fits my experience. I believe that the B lesions are worse than the A lesions, but this is still at the stage of hypothesis. We should try to agree on the factual bases for making decisions, and these are not very many. When considering just the parenchymal cell lesions, starting with the classification which we discussed previously and adding non-neoplastic nodules which I have sub-divided into non-hyperplastic nodules and hyperplastic nodules, we then have liver cell adenomas and hepatocellular carcinomas which we have divided into four types: (*1*) Non-metastasising; (*2*) Locally invasive; (*3*) With emboli in lungs, and (*4*) With metastases.

Chapter 4

Carcinogenesis and Cell Proliferation in Mouse Liver with Dimethylnitrosamine

SHOZO TAKAYAMA

Cancer Institute,
1-37-1 Kami-Ikebukuro,
Tohsima-Ku, Tokyo 170
(Japan)

INTRODUCTION

Several strains of mice have consistently been shown to develop liver tumours as well as lung tumours when adult mice received a low concentration of dimethylnitrosamine (DMN) in their drinking water or diet for a long period. The liver tumours were predominantly haemangiosarcomas (SCHMÄHL *et al.*, 1963; TAKAYAMA AND OOTA, 1963, 1965; TOTH *et al.*, 1964; TERRACINI *et al.*, 1966; CLAPP AND TOYA SR., 1970; VESSELINOVITCH, 1969; OTSUKA AND KUWAHARA, 1971; CLAPP AND CRAIG, 1967; CLAPP *et al.*, 1968, 1971).

After a single injection or short term administration of a fairly high concentration of DMN to newborn or young adult mice, the main sites of tumour formation were the lung, kidney and liver. The most common types of liver tumours were, however, liver cell adenomas and liver cell carcinomas (TERRACINI *et al.*, 1966; TOTH *et al.*, 1964). Induction of vascular neoplasms by oral administration of DMN and its derivatives was described by SCHMÄHL AND PREUSSMANN (1959) and LESCH *et al.* (1967) in rats. HERROLD (1967) and OTSUKA AND KUWAHARA (1971) reported on the histogenesis of liver neoplasms induced with DMN in hamsters. Based on their observation of the series of lesions they concluded that haemangioendothelial sarcoma started from the simple proliferation of reticuloendothelial cells which developed into a neoplasm with the characteristic histological picture of haemangioendothelial sarcoma.

Using isotopically labelled DMN, several investigators have concluded that methylation of nucleic acids is important for the initiation of carcinogenesis and that the susceptibility of various organs to the formation of tumours depends on the amount of N^7-methylguanine produced. However, in their experiments, the doses of [3]H- or ^{14}C-labelled DMN were high resulting in widespread centrilobular necrosis of the liver (LAWLEY *et al.*, 1968; LEE *et al.*, 1964; MAGEE AND FARBER, 1962; SWANN AND MAGEE, 1968).

In view of the importance of correlating the information on the cellular origin in experimental liver neoplasms with the chemical interactions, the present studies were initiated. First the histogenesis of haemangiomas induced by DMN in ICR mice is described with emphasis on histological and autoradiographical observation. Secondly the formation of N^7-methylguanine in nucleic acid of the liver, lung and kidney under conditions similar to those inducing liver carcinomas with [^{3}H]DMN.

METHODS

In the present experiments, 8-week-old male ICR mice were used. For the study of the histogenesis of the neoplasm, mice were given a diet of 50 ppm DMN and killed after 1, 3 and 7 days and 3, 5, 7, 10, 15, 25 and 35 weeks on the diet. Two mice were killed at each time interval; 1 h before killing each mouse was given 100 μCi of [^{3}H]thymidine (specific activity 6·7 Ci/mmole) intraperitoneally. Kodak AR 10 stripping film was used for the autoradiographic procedures.

For differential counting of cell types in the liver sections, a reticle delimiting a square field was placed in one of the oculars of a binocular microscope. Differential counts of the following cell types were made; liver parenchymal cells, bile-duct cells, sinusoidal endothelial cells, cells of the blood vessel walls, and cells of connective tissue. At least 5000 nuclei were examined for each animal.

The present experiment was undertaken primarily to study N^7-methylguanine formation in the nucleic acids of mouse liver, lung, and kidney under conditions similar to those inducing liver carcinogenesis with [^{3}H]DMN.

To study the incorporation of labelled DMN the mice were given 10 ppm of [^{3}H]DMN solution as drinking water *ad libitum* and killed at 1, 2, 3, 5, 7, 10, 14, 21 and 30 days. Two mice were killed at each time interval. Preparation of nuclear DNA and cytoplasmic RNA from the livers, lungs and kidneys has been described previously (NEMOTO AND TAKAYAMA, 1973).

RESULTS

Pathological findings

After 3 and 7 days on the DMN diet (50 ppm) the most conspicuous morphological findings were vacuolation of cytoplasm near the central vein. The nuclei were swollen, pale and irregular in outline. The periphery of the lobules was unaffected.

After 3 to 7 weeks coagulative necrosis was observed in the centrilobular zone (Fig. 1). More or less extensive haemorrhagic changes were associated with parenchymal cell necrosis, and the resorption of necrotic foci was followed by small, blood-filled cysts. These blood cysts were delimited by parenchymal cells and lacked distinct endothelial lining cells.

In mice killed at 20 weeks, enlarged liver parenchymal cells were observed. The cells varied in size, some containing a large nucleus with coarse chromatin and prominent nucleoli. The sinusoid endothelium was prominent.

A remarkable sinusoidal cell proliferation was observed in animals killed in the

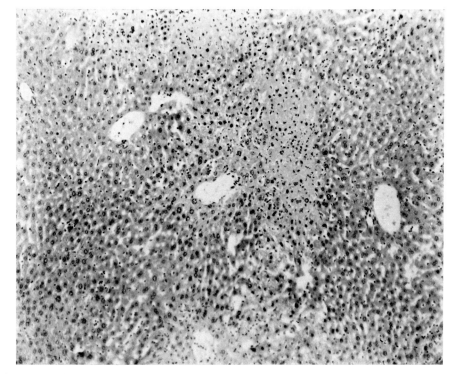

Fig. 1. Necrosis of the centrilobular zone of the liver. H and E ×100.

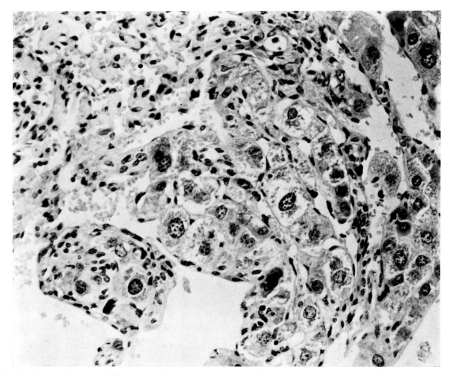

Fig. 2. Liver of mouse killed after 25 weeks of DMN diet showing sinusoidal endothelial cell proliferation and polymorphism of the liver parenchymal cells. H and E ×200.

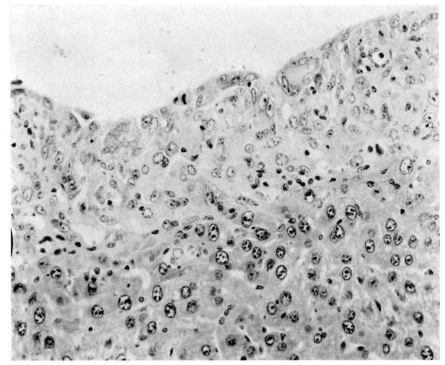

Fig. 3. Liver of mouse killed after 25 weeks of DMN diet showing focal proliferation of endothelial cells. Mitotic figures are present. H and E ×200.

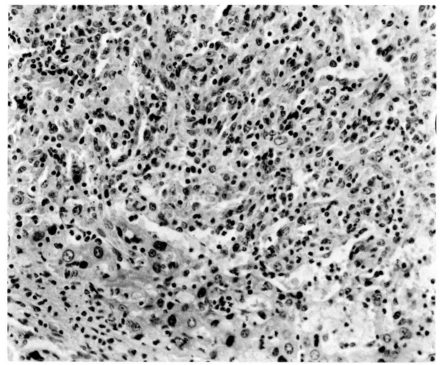

Fig. 4. Liver of mouse killed after 35 weeks of DMN diet showing a haemangiomatous neoplasm of the liver. Irregular vascular clefts are evident in proliferating spindle-shaped or oval cells. H and E ×200.

25th week. The liver parenchymal cells showed polymorphism (Fig. 2). The boundary of the cells was poorly defined and basophilic nuclei were prominent. The liver cords were disrupted, leading to the development of irregular vascular spaces. The enlarged sinusoidal endothelium lay directly adjacent to the liver parenchymal cells. There were some areas in which focal proliferation of sinusoidal cells was observed (Fig. 3). In such areas the liver parenchymal cells had disappeared.

In animals killed after 35 weeks, haemangiomatous neoplasm was found. It was recognized as dark brownish, or cystic nodules in the liver. The tumour consisted of densely proliferating spindle cells with occasional arrangements forming cleft-like spaces (Fig. 4). No metastases were found.

Autoradiographical findings

The lesions were found diffusely scattered throughout the liver lobules. To calculate the percentage of labelled cells, all the cells were counted in a certain square (about 3 mm^2) selected to calculate the proportion of each cell to warrant an unbiased cell count. In this experiment, more labelled cells were found among the sinusoidal cells than in the liver parenchymal cells throughout the experiment (Table I).

In control mice, 0·19% of the liver parenchymal cells, 0·67% of the sinusoidal cells, 0·19% of the bile duct cells, 0% of cells of the major blood vessel walls, and 0% of cells of the connective tissue cells were labelled. However, one day after feeding DMN 3·5% of the sinusoidal cells were labelled. This might suggest a transient increase of metabolism in the liver. After 3 days on the DMN diet, however, the number of labelled sinusoidal cells decreased rapidly, probably due to the acute toxic effects of

TABLE I

LABELLING INDEX OF VARIOUS LIVER CELLS IN MICE FED DMN

Time of diet	Cell types in the liver				
	Liver parenchymal cells	Sinusoidal endothelial cells	Cells of bile ducts	Cells of blood vessel walls	Cells of connective tissue
Control	0.19	0.67	0.19	0	0
1 day	0.32	3.58	0	0.88	0
3 days	0.09	2.33	0.72	0	0
1 week	0.80	3.21	0.30	1.55	0
3 weeks	0.76	2.21	0.48	0.55	0
5 weeks	0.56	3.03	0	0.63	0
7 weeks	0.51	3.51	0	1.22	0
10 weeks	0.97	4.03	0.30	1.43	0
15 weeks	0.20	2.42	0	0	0
20 weeks	0.19	2.58	0	0	0
25 weeks	0.12	2.23	0	0	0
35 weeks	1.05	3.86	0	1.34	0

TABLE II

NUMERICAL PROPORTION OF CELL TYPES IN THE LIVER OF MICE FED DMN

Time of diet	Percent distribution of cell types ($\pm$ S.D.)				
	Liver cells	Sinusoidal endothelial cells	Cells of bile duct	Cells of blood vessel walls	Cells of connective tissue
Control	61.68 $\pm$ 6.42	32.99 $\pm$ 5.30	1.62 $\pm$ 3.24	3.21 $\pm$ 1.48	0.51 $\pm$ 1.49
1 day	64.23 $\pm$ 5.38	29.94 $\pm$ 5.98	2.19 $\pm$ 4.24	3.45 $\pm$ 1.55	0.19 $\pm$ 0.58
3 days	67.61 $\pm$ 5.10	29.78 $\pm$ 4.80	0.84 $\pm$ 2.54	1.75 $\pm$ 1.95	0.20 $\pm$ 1.08
1 week	62.74 $\pm$ 7.03	33.22 $\pm$ 9.72	1.24 $\pm$ 2.15	2.07 $\pm$ 2.99	0.89 $\pm$ 1.85
3 weeks	42.79 $\pm$ 10.18	51.22 $\pm$ 10.86	2.01 $\pm$ 5.60	3.76 $\pm$ 3.91	0.22 $\pm$ 1.05
5 weeks	58.26 $\pm$ 5.34	38.62 $\pm$ 4.95	0.73 $\pm$ 1.87	1.88 $\pm$ 2.43	0.52 $\pm$ 1.23
7 weeks	56.90 $\pm$ 4.50	41.40 $\pm$ 5.13	0.53 $\pm$ 1.11	1.14 $\pm$ 2.12	0.03 $\pm$ 0.18
10 weeks	52.82 $\pm$ 6.43	44.52 $\pm$ 6.42	0.91 $\pm$ 2.34	1.63 $\pm$ 2.59	0.12 $\pm$ 0.47
15 weeks	49.79 $\pm$ 12.34	47.90 $\pm$ 11.54	1.28 $\pm$ 3.15	1.99 $\pm$ 3.58	0.04 $\pm$ 0.23
20 weeks	63.87 $\pm$ 6.29	32.33 $\pm$ 3.82	1.91 $\pm$ 6.20	1.67 $\pm$ 2.52	0.22 $\pm$ 0.99
25 weeks	63.83 $\pm$ 4.13	33.56 $\pm$ 3.61	0.88 $\pm$ 1.68	1.73 $\pm$ 2.06	0
35 weeks	62.81 $\pm$ 5.99	34.71 $\pm$ 4.69	0.81 $\pm$ 2.28	1.59 $\pm$ 1.87	0.07 $\pm$ 0.33

DMN on the liver. After 1 week, the number of labelled sinusoidal cells again increased. In 3 weeks, values again decreased to the level similar to that on the third day. A gradual increase was subsequently found and the percentage of labelled sinusoidal cells reached 4·03% in the 10th week following DMN feeding.

The tendency of increase or decrease in the number of labelled cells among the liver parenchymal cells paralleled the behaviour of the sinusoidal cells.

In animals killed in the advanced stage, focal proliferation of the sinusoidal endothelial cells was found. When only such field was chosen, the proportion of the number of labelled cells increased to 8·02%. Haemangiomatous lesions were found in a mouse killed in the 35th week. The percentage of labelled cells in the tumour alone was 9·67%.

Kinetics of incorporation of radioactivity into the nucleic acids of various organs

The labelling of liver RNA during the experimental period reached a plateau within 2 weeks. However, at the end of the period it decreased, and the specific activity of RNA after 30 days was less than that after 21 days. The labelling of RNA in the lung and kidney was negligible after 3 days and only slight after one week. Then the labelling in the lung RNA increased, reaching the same level as that in the liver after 2 weeks. The specific activity of the kidney RNA increased gradually. RNA in the lung and kidney had a higher specific activity than that in the liver after 30 days. As shown in Fig. 5 the kinetic pattern of labelling the nuclear DNA was similar to that of cytoplasmic RNA.

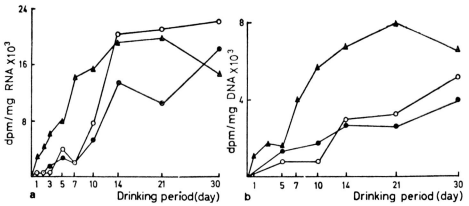

Fig. 5a and b. Kinetics of labelling of nuclear DNA and cytoplasmic RNA. Mice were given 6·8–9·7 μCi of [³H]DMN per day in the drinking water and killed at the times indicated. The nuclear and cytoplasmic fractions of the liver, lungs and kidneys were isolated. DNA was prepared from the nuclear fraction and RNA from the cytoplasmic fraction as described in the text. (a), Cytoplasmic RNA: (b), Nuclear DNA; ▲———▲, liver; ○– – –○, lungs; ●———●, kidneys. Each point represents the average of values in 2 animals. (NEMOTO AND TAKAYAMA, 1973).

Formation of N^7-methylguanine in nucleic acids

MAGEE AND FARBER (1962), SWANN AND MAGEE (1968), LAWLEY *et al.* (1968) and MURAMATSU *et al.* (1972) showed that after a single injection of isotopically labelled DMN, radioactivity was chiefly associated with N^7-methylguanine. To examine what proportion of guanine residues were methylated in this experiment, nucleic acids were hydrolysed and analysed using a Dowex 50 column.

The elution patterns of hydrolysates of liver DNA shown in Fig. 6 indicate that after 7 days almost all the radioactivity was eluted in a peak between those of guanine and adenine identified as N^7-methylguanine. After 10 to 21 days, radioactivity was also found in minor peaks in the void volume, and in the peaks of guanine and adenine. After 30 days, radioactivity was found in the peaks of guanine and adenine, *i.e.* in the normal constituents of nucleic acid.

The alteration in the pattern of cytoplasmic RNA was more remarkable. Almost all the radioactivity was associated with the N^7-methylguanine fraction, but the guanine and adenine fractions also had some radioactivity even after one day (Fig. 7).

The ratio of the sum of radioactivity in the guanine and adenine fraction to that in the N^7-methylguanine fraction gradually increased, and after 30 days, the total radioactivity eluted in the guanine and adenine fractions was more than that in the N^7-methylguanine fraction.

Methylation of guanine residues in nucleic acids

Acid hydrolysates of nucleic acids were fractionated by ion-exchange chromatography, and then the number of molecules of guanine and N^7-methylguanine in each

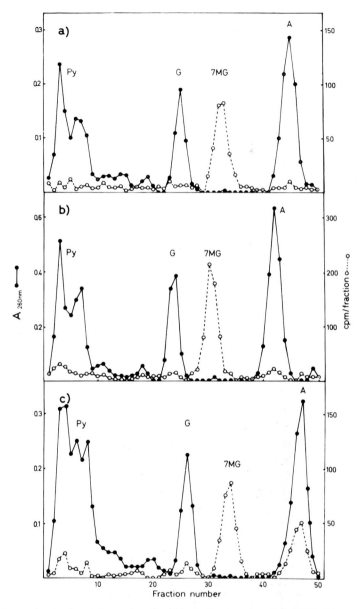

Fig. 6a–c. Ion-exchange chromatography of acid hydrolysates of nuclear DNA. Liver nuclear DNA was hydrolyzed by treatment with 1 N HCl at 100° for 1 h. The hydrolysate was applied to a Dowex 50 column (1·0×20 cm) and developed with a linear gradient of 1–4 N HCl. Py, pyrimidine nucleotide; G, guanine; 7MG, N^7-methylguanine; A, adenine. (a), Nuclear DNA after 7 days; (b), DNA after 10 days; (c), DNA after 30 days. (NEMOTO AND TAKAYAMA, 1973)

fraction was calculated from the absorbance at 260 nm and from the radioactivity, respectively (Tables III and IV).

From the first to the 21st day, the proportion of guanine residues methylated in the liver DNA increased gradually, and about 0·1 % of the guanine residues were

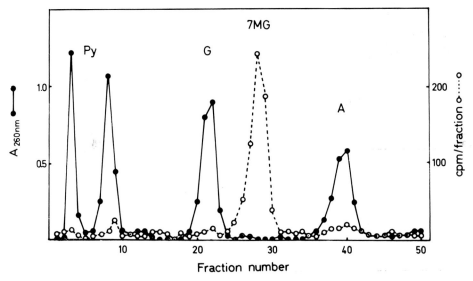

Fig. 7. Ion-exchange chromatography of acid hydrolysate of liver cytoplasmic RNA after 1 day. (NEMOTO AND TAKAYAMA, 1973)

methylated at the N-7 position after 21 days. But after 30 days, the proportion decreased to less than half that found at 21 days, although there was no significant change in the volume of water imbibed during the experimental period. The same changes were observed in the liver cytoplasmic RNA. Also, in the liver RNA, the amount of N^7-methylguanine after 30 days was only about two-thirds of that after 21 days. In the first 7 days RNA in the lung and kidney could not be analyzed because the labelling was too low. However, the proportion of guanine residues methylated in the kidney RNA increased with time and after 30 days the percentage of N^7-methylguanine to total guanine in the kidney RNA was about half that in the liver RNA. In the lung RNA, the percentage gradually increased, and was a quarter of that in the liver RNA after 30 days.

TABLE III

METHYLATION OF THE N-7 POSITION OF GUANINE OF NUCLEAR DNA IN LIVER

Acid hydrolysates of nuclear DNA were fractionated and the proportion of guanine residues methylated was calculated from the absorbance of the guanine fraction and the radioactivity of the N^7-methylguanine fraction as described in the previous report. (NEMOTO AND TAKAYAMA, 1973)

Drinking period (day)	Guanine residues methylated (% of total)
5	0.022
7	0.046
10	0.057
14	0.073
21	0.098
30	0.041

TABLE IV

METHYLATION TO THE *N*-7 POSITION OF GUANINE OF CYTOPLASMIC RNA IN VARIOUS ORGANS

Results were calculated as for nuclear DNA. The values for liver RNA after 1 and 2 days were obtained for total cytoplasmic RNA. (NEMOTO AND TAKAYAMA, 1973)

Drinking period (day)	Guanine residues methylated (% of total)			Lung	Kidney
	Liver				
	28S	18S	~4S		
1		0.025		—	—
2		0.034		—	—
5	0.054	0.050	0.054		—
7	0.065	0.072	0.082	—	—
10	0.081	0.091	0.064	0.008	0.008
14	0.106	0.123	0.141	0.010	0.010
21	0.129	0.130	0.125	0.017	0.027
30	0.077	0.083	0.085	0.018	0.044

The proportion of guanine residues methylated was 1·6–2·5 times higher in RNA than in DNA. The proportions of guanine residues methylated in 28S, 18S and ~4S RNA of liver cytoplasm were similar throughout the experiment.

DISCUSSION

DMN acts as a toxic substance producing necrosis in mouse liver. Occurrence of incorporation of [^{3}H]thymidine into the sinusoidal endothelial cells was seen as early as after 1 day. This proliferation continued for many weeks.

Among the labelled cells, there was a high proportion of sinusoidal endothelial cells. Although the numerical proportion of liver parenchymal cells and sinusoidal cells was approximately 50:50 in the liver 10 weeks after DMN administrations, the labelling index was 0·97% and 4·03% respectively (Tables I and II), which might indicate the active reaction of sinusoidal endothelial cells with DMN.

The above findings indicate that haemangioma of the liver induced by DMN develops from the proliferation of sinusoidal endothelial cells. Our present experimental results are similar to the hamster experiment reported by HERROLD (1967) and OTSUKA AND KUWAHARA (1971), suggesting that the development of the neoplasm was the result of the proliferation of sinusoidal endothelial cells.

We have also demonstrated that liver nucleic acids were preferentially labelled in the initial stages while labelling of those of the lung and kidney gradually increased, reaching almost the same level as that of the liver nucleic acids after 30 days. However, throughout this period, methylation of the N-7 position of guanine in liver nucleic acids was consistently higher than that of either kidney or lung.

Paralleling this biochemical study, a further carcinogenicity study was also performed. The mice were given drinking water containing 5 ppm DMN for the first

30 days and killed after a further 335 days. Tumours were observed in 90% of the lungs, 20% of the livers, and 10% of the kidneys (unpublished data).

Small amounts of abnormal methylated bases such as O^7-methylguanine and [^{3}H]methyladenine may also have been formed under the experimental conditions, as in the chromatography of acid hydrolysates of nucleic acids several small peaks of radioactivity other than those of N^7-methylguanine and major constituents of nucleic acid, were always detected. During the experimental period labelling of guanine and adenine gradually increased, finally exceeding that of N^7-methylguanine.

If it is assumed that most of the incorporation of labelled DMN is into hepatocyte nucleic acids, it would appear that the significance of the binding of DMN to cellular macromolecules under conditions inducing vascular tumours should be re-evaluated.

These results also indicate that there is no definite correlation between tumour incidence in liver, lung and kidney and the amount of N^7-methylguanine formation.

REFERENCES

CLAPP, N. K., AND CRAIG, A. S. (1967) Carcinogenic effects of diethylnitrosamine in RF mice. *J. Natl. Cancer Inst.*, 39: 903.

CLAPP, N. K., CRAIG, A. W., AND TOYA SR., R. E. (1968) Pulmonary and hepatic oncogenesis during treatment of male RF mice with dimethylnitrosamine. *J. Natl. Cancer Inst.*, 41: 1213.

CLAPP, N. K., AND TOYA SR., R. E. (1970) Effect of cumulative dose and dose rate on dimethyl-nitrosamine oncogenesis in RF mice. *J. Natl. Cancer Inst.*, 45: 495.

CLAPP, N. K., TYNDALL, R. L. AND OTTEN, J. A. (1971) Differences in tumour types and organ susceptibility in BALB/c and RF mice following dimethylnitrosamine and diethylnitrosamine. *Cancer Res.*, 31: 196.

HERROLD, K. M. (1967) Histogenesis of malignant liver tumours induced by dimethylnitrosamine. An experimental study in Syrian hamsters. *J. Natl. Cancer Inst.*, 39: 1099.

LAWLEY, P. D., BROOKES, P., MAGEE, P. N., CRADDOCK, V. M., AND SWANN, P. F. (1968) Methylated bases in liver nucleic acids from rats treated with dimethylnitrosamine. *Biochim. biophys. Acta*, 157: 646.

LEE, K. Y., LIJINSKY, W., AND MAGEE, P. N. (1964) Methylation of ribonucleic acids of liver and other organs in different species treated with C^{14}- and H^3-dimethylnitrosamine *in vivo*. *J. Natl. Cancer Inst.*, 32: 65.

LESCH, R., MEINHARDT, K., AND OEHLERT, W. (1967) Lichtmikroskopische und autoradiographische Befunde bei der Cancerisierung der Rattenleber mit Methyl-Allyl-Nitrosamin. *Z. Krebsforsch.*, 70: 267.

MAGEE, P. N., AND FARBER, E. (1962) Toxic liver injury and carcinogenesis; methylation of rat liver nucleic acid by dimethylnitrosamine *in vivo*. *Biochem. J.*, 83; 114.

MURAMATSU, M., AZAMA, Y., NEMOTO, N., AND TAKAYAMA, S. (1972) Methylation of nuclear and cytoplasmic RNA of mouse liver with dimethylnitrosamine-^{3}H. *Cancer Res.*, 32: 702.

NEMOTO, N., AND TAKAYAMA, S. (1973) Formation of N^7-methylguanine in nuclear DNA and cytoplasmic RNA in mice on continuous oral administration of dimethylnitrosamine-^{3}H solution. *Z. Krebsforsch.*, 80: 113.

SWANN, P. F., AND MAGEE, P. N. (1968) Nitrosamine-induced carcinogenesis. The alkylation of nucleic acids of the rat by N-methyl-N-nitrosourea, dimethylnitrosamine, dimethyl sulphate and methyl methanesulphonate. *Biochem. J.*, 110: 39.

OTSUKA, H., AND KUWAHARA, A. (1971) Hemangiomatous lesions of mice treated with nitroso-dimethylamine. *Gann*, 62: 147.

SCHMÄHL, D., AND PREUSSMANN, R. (1959) Cancerogene Wirkung von Nitrosodimethylamin bei Ratten. *Naturwissensch.*, 46: 175.

SCHMÄHL, D., PREUSSMANN, R., THOMAS, C., AND KÖNIG, J. (1963) Versuche zur Krebserzeugung mit Diäthylnitrosamin bei Mäusen. *Naturwissensch.*, 50: 407.

TAKAYAMA, S., AND OOTA, K. (1963) Malignant tumors induced in mice fed with N-nitrosodimethyl-amine. *Gann*, 54: 465.

TAKAYAMA, S., AND OOTA, K. (1965) Induction of malignant tumors in various strains of mice by oral administration of N-nitrosodimethylamine and N-nitrosodiethylamine. *Gann*, 56: 189.

TERRACINI, PLESTRO G., RAMELLA GIGLIARDI, M., AND MONTESANO, R. (1966) Carcinogenicity of dimethylnitrosamine in Swiss mice. *Brit. J. Cancer*, 20: 871.

TOTH, B., MAGEE, P. N., AND SHUBIK, P. (1964) Carcinogenesis study with dimethylnitrosamine administered orally to adult and subcutaneously to newborn BALB/c mice. *Cancer Res.*, 24: 1712.

VESSELINOVITCH, S. D. (1969) The sex-dependent difference in the development of liver tumors in mice administered dimethylnitrosamine. *Cancer Res.*, 29: 1024.

DISCUSSION

BUTLER. May we be clear as to the incidence of tumours and the histological type at the doses of 5 and 50 ppm DMN?

TAKAYAMA. Five ppm DMN for 30 days resulted in an eventual incidence of 20% hepatic neoplasms at 1 year. 60% of these were parenchymal cell and 40% were vascular. At 50 ppm all the tumours were vascular and were present at 35 weeks. At 50 ppm DMN in the diet, many animals died at an early age with ascites. However, the survivors had vascular tumours in the liver as well as kidney and lung. In the earlier stages when the animals died from ascites there was evidence of centrilobular hepatic necrosis, but we did not do special stains to demonstrate the veno-occlusive disease that has been reported following DMN treatment.

LAQUEUR. Proliferation of the reticulo-endothelial cells lining the sinusoids is becoming an acute problem and is assuming a great importance. It has been known for at least ten years that diethyl-nitrosamine given to hamsters produces a proliferation of the endothelium of the sinusoids. We also described a similar phenomenon when we investigated methylazoxymethanol, the aglycone of cycasin. Recently, vascular lesions have been found in the liver of people following exposure to vinyl chloride monomer. In all these situations there are proliferative changes of the reticulo-endothelial cells either adjacent to an angiosarcoma or at least occurring in the same liver as angiosarcoma which may have been induced by these compounds. A variant of this which I have seen is a reticulum cell sarcoma. In other systems, proliferation of the reticulo-endothelial cells of the sinusoids has been seen. These observations in both laboratory animals and in man fit very well with the studies of Dr. TAKAYAMA.

GRASSO. To what extent do you consider cell proliferation is necessary to precede cancer in the liver as there is evidence in the system of subcutaneous sarcomas that there was a preceding proliferative response?

BUTLER. When considering vascular neoplasia it is interesting to consider the role of proliferating granulation tissue. Dr. Takayama described areas of necrosis which will elicit a granulation tissue reaction. Does this play any role in the development of angiosarcoma? There is one small piece of evidence in the rat that angiosarcoma can arise from granulation tissue. Dr. CRADDOCK (1971, *J. Natl. Cancer Inst.*, 47: 889) studied the effect of partial hepatectomy on DMN-induced hepatic carcinogenesis and found angiosarcoma derived from the stump as well as hepatic carcinoma.

LAQUEUR. During the time that the fibrosis occurs there is some chronic inflammatory reaction but in the stages that I have seen it did not suggest granulation tissue.

TAKAYAMA. The fibrosis and necrosis appear to be strain-dependent in the mouse while angio-sarcoma appears to be independent of fibrosis. There appears to be no sex difference in the incidence of vascular tumours while there is a sex difference in parenchymal cell tumours.

BUTLER. Is there any evidence in the mouse of the cellular events which may precede hepatocellular carcinoma in the rat? An interpretation of the development of the vascular lesion seen in the mouse could be that it is not a multi-stage process. In the rat there is conflicting evidence. There is evidence that hepatic carcinoma in the rat may in some instances be preceded by a phase of hyperplasia, but there is no good evidence that there needs to be a preceding cirrhosis.

GRASSO. In the rat there is evidence in DMN-induced tumours that there is a dose which does not result in any of the pathological processes mentioned prior to the induction of carcinoma. At between 10–15 ppm DMN tumours may be induced at 350 to 400 days, and sequential studies fail to reveal any prior necrosis or fibrosis. However, in the mouse there is very little published evidence.

The importance of preceding tissue injury in the development of hepatic nodular lesions has been studied utilizing CCl_4 and $CHCl_3$. Both compounds produce extensive necrosis in the hepatic centrilobular areas as well as hepatoma [ESCHENBRENNER AND MILLER (1945) J. Natl. Cancer Inst., 5: 251; ESCHENBRENNER AND MILLER (1946) J. Natl. Cancer Inst., 6: 325]. A dose–response study using chloroform showed that there is a sudden drop in the incidence of tumours in female mice between the second highest dose and the next lower dose. The study of the histological changes preceding CCl_4-induced hepatoma received detailed attention in earlier studies by EDWARDS AND DALTON (1942, J. Natl. Cancer Inst., 3: 19). Sequential studies on mice receiving 0·04 ml of CCl_4 twice or three times weekly for up to 23–58 doses revealed that after the first dose there was extensive necrosis of the liver involving the central one-third to one-half of the lobule. In about 2 weeks the centrilobular areas contained some necrotic debris and dilated sinusoids without viable cells. The necrotic process gradually spread to the portal tracts and there was also an accompanying increase in connective tissue round the central zones. At this stage restoration of the parenchymal cells was evident and this progressed as the experiment proceeded. The original architecture of the liver was grossly disturbed so that, eventually, the regenerated parenchymal was divided by connective tissue into discrete lobules. Of the treated mice that had received less than 23 injections and were allowed to live till the end of the experiment (12 months after first treatment) none developed hepatomas, whereas the incidence of these lesions in mice that had received between 25–58 doses varied from 60–89% depending on the strain of mice used. The primary tumours were transplantable in mice of the same strain.

ESCHENBRENNER AND MILLER (1946, J. Natl. Cancer Inst., 6: 325) investigated the dose–response relationship to tumour formation by repeated CCl_4 administration, and the effect of increasing the time interval between successive doses on tumour formation, and demonstrated that spacing the dose levels has as much influence on tumour induction as increasing the dose. In order to explain this, the authors postulated that the tumours arose as a result of repeated cycles of necrosis and regeneration which were optimum when an interval of 3–4 days was allowed. This biological situation has a parallel in the evolution of sarcoma in rats by repeated injections of surfactants. If injections are stopped before the 4th month no tumours develop, whereas if they are carried on up to the 6th and 7th month a substantial number of rats develop local sarcomas [HOOSON et al. (1973) Brit. J. Cancer, 27: 230].

Another point of interest is that, in the mouse, the few dose-related studies carried out indicate that the response to carcinogens seems to differ considerably from the results obtained with CCl_4 and $CHCl_3$. Thus, reducing the dose level did not reduce markedly the number of malignant tumours with DMN or DEN. Thus, there are indications that the mouse liver-nodule could result from successive episodes of tissue injury and repair as well as a process of so-called "chemical carcinogenesis", and on this basis one cannot accept its induction, assuming that it is a cancer, as unequivocal evidence of carcinogenicity.

A possible mechanism for this may be that focal nodular lesions, which are not necessarily neoplastic, may have a different blood supply and microsomal enzymes with a resulting different pattern of metabolism of the toxic compound with the formation of abnormal metabolic intermediaries which would not occur in normal parenchymal cells. If this is correct and the dose level is reduced so that the focal response is absent, tumours will not be induced. To study this we are using dimethylnitrosamine and saffrole.

P. M. NEWBERNE. It is being suggested that necrosis is a necessary precursor of parenchymal cell neoplasia? Or am I interpreting the situation correctly by saying that if you injure a liver and superimpose a compound on it that you may get a false positive by virtue of the injury to the liver?

GRASSO. Loosely, yes, but I have no good idea what type of injury is required. However, there appear to be two groups of compounds; one produces a gradual dose response to tumour induction while the other result is a sharp step-like response related to injury. It is a great step forward if you consider those with the step-like response resulting from hepatotoxicity as a phenomenon of toxicity and not carcinogenic in terms of carcinogenic hazard. One is then in the realm of reason. If you call a compound carcinogenic, one is in the realm of emotion. I am not suggesting that the compound is not a carcinogen by definition but that it arises by a different mechanism.

PHILP. ESCHENBRENNER's study quoted by Dr. GRASSO shows clearly that if one uses a compound that causes hepatic injury and continue to dose the compound, it is being added to a very abnormal system. When fibrosis and necrosis are reduced, one is unlikely to get tumours. This is worth studying further.

BUTLER. Possibly as all hepatocarcinogens are hepatotoxic one is dealing with two dose response curves of two separate phenomena. It would then be incorrect to suggest that the carcinomas in the presence of injury were false positive results.

PHILP. The suggestion of false positives clouds the issue. I think that it has been demonstrated that there are different mechanisms by which carcinomas are induced. If an end point is to predict that a hepatotoxic compound is a carcinogen for man of the same potency as other carcinogens, such as the nitrosamines, in effect the result is a false positive.

GRASSO. My feeling would be that with compounds which produce extensive injury prior to the development of carcinoma, there must be a dose where one is reasonably safe in not inducing carcinomas. However, with the group where gross damage does not precede the neoplasm one is less certain of a safe level.

REUBER. Returning to BUTLER's question concerning hyperplasia. I have done sequential killing in mice, and unpublished data would indicate a progression from hyperplasia to neoplasia. When we ask whether a carcinoma develops from a previous lesion, I have no doubt that they all do, but we have chosen models where they develop slowly enough for us to follow them. Where a rapidly growing neoplasm is induced, the stages may be missed. I would consider that the changes in the mouse parallel those of the rat.

ROE. Unless one actually does the experiment in the mouse, one cannot assume that they are the same as the rat. There are some parallels, but in my experience the process appears to be different.

GRASSO. I would agree with Dr. ROE that because one sees nodules at laparotomy and later carcinoma that one cannot conclude that one lesion develops from the other. It is possible that the original nodule was a carcinoma at the time it was observed.

ROE. When one sees four different lesions in the liver it is not possible to say that one progresses to another. At other sites one has seen lesions which in the main are not malignant but which contain areas of more bizarre histology. This is the best evidence available at present of progression of lesions. On occasion we have seen this in the liver.

REUBER. I have seen areas of hyperplasia within which malignant cells are present. My definition of an adenoma is a benign lesion which should not become malignant, while hyperplasia will progress to malignant neoplasia. I think most lesions one sees in the mouse liver are either hyperplasia or malignant neoplasia, while benign tumours are rare.

BUTLER. Do you consider nodular hyperplasia an inevitable precursor of malignant neoplasia?

REUBER. Yes, if the animal lives long enough.

ROE. We appear to have very little agreement on this matter as I consider that I have seen benign neoplasia progress to malignant neoplasia, but I have never seen nodular hyperplasia in the mouse liver. However, I have seen nodules but have no evidence that they are hyperplastic.

HOLLANDER. Is it possible to look at a liver with multiple nodules and say which have metastasised? As I have mentioned, I tried to do this in a series of liver tumours in mice, but I was unable to identify which had metastasised. I feel that there is a progression of hyperplasia to malignancy, but I do not have the evidence for this.

TAKAYAMA. We treated a series of CDF$_1$ mice with benzenehexachloride (a-BHC) 500 ppm for 24 weeks. At that time 50 male and 50 female mice were killed. The incidence of nodules was 100% in the males and 80–90% in the females. A further group of animals of the same size were returned to the normal diet and killed after a further 24 weeks, at which time the incidence of nodules was 53% in the males and 40% in the females. This indicates that these nodules regress. If the a-BHC is given for 36 weeks and then the animals returned to normal diet, the lesions appear to regress more slowly.

REUBER. I have performed similar experiments with acetylamino fluorine and failed to find regression.

P. M. NEWBERNE. I am as appalled now as I was 6 months ago when I started to read up on this subject, as to how little we know about the mouse compared with the rat. One sees nodules but there is little agreement as to their nature. Morphology alone does not appear to be a sufficient guide to accurate diagnosis; it is obviously necessary to consider the biology of the lesion.

BUTLER. How do you reconcile the biochemical data of the incorporation into nucleic acids with the histological evidence of vascular neoplasia?

GRASSO. If the presence of N^7-methylguanine is relevant to carcinogenesis it may not be possible to reconcile these observations.

TAKAYAMA. Most biochemical studies are the result of a single administration of the compound but there is little evidence of what happens during carcinogenesis leading to liver tumours. Therefore I endeavoured to investigate conditions leading to carcinoma. We found a number of peaks in the adenine and guanine fractions which are normal constituents. We also found O-6-methylguanine and N-3-methyladenine. It is possible that these minor peaks produce some mutagenic response.

Chapter 5

The Natural History of Hepatic Parenchymal Nodule Formation in a Colony of C57BL Mice with Reference to the Effect of Diet

J. B. M. GELLATLY

Unilever Research Laboratory Colworth/Welwyn, Colworth House, Sharnbrook, Bedford (Great Britain)

INTRODUCTION

Published work on the influence of nutrition on the genesis of tumours and their growth is extensive and is the subject of major reviews by TANNENBAUM (1953), TANNENBAUM AND SILVERSTONE (1953), COWDRY (1955), HAVEN AND BLOOR (1956), HENDERSON AND LEPAGE (1959), MCCOY (1959), WHITE (1961) and MURRAY *et al.* (1968). Information relevant to hepatomas in mice is, however, somewhat scanty.

The effects of a reduction in calorie intake by under-feeding, intermittent fasting or calorie restriction are well documented. MORESCHI (1909) reported that sarcoma transplantation in mice was more difficult in dietary restricted animals and that tumour growth was roughly proportional to food intake. Subsequently, MCCAY *et al.* (1939) demonstrated that the incidence of spontaneous tumours in rats was reduced by a moderate degree of under-feeding. Thereafter, several investigators studied the effect of under-feeding on the partial or total inhibition of the formation of spontaneous and induced tumours including spontaneous hepatomas in mice (TANNENBAUM AND SILVERSTONE, 1949). As TANNENBAUM (1953) has pointed out, however, there are no satisfactory means of ascribing "normal" values for either caloric intake or body weight in experimental animals since the effects of age, strain, dietary composition, method of housing and amount of voluntary exercise must be considered. In many laboratories, mice fed *ad libitum* often attain relatively high body weights, with large fat depots and clinical obesity. Calorie restriction of 50–75% not only reduces body weight but also produces mice which are sleek, active and of longer life span; reduced tumour incidence and the later development of tumours in such animals are certainly not a consequence of increased debility or premature death (TANNENBAUM, 1940). Indeed, it may be probable that the calorie restricted animal, by virtue of longevity and improved health is more "normal" than its obese counterpart.

Colworth C57BL colony

In this paper, the natural history of one lesion as it occurs in the Colworth C57Black (C57BL) colony will be reviewed. This colony was established in 1959 from a nucleus of three pairs of mice with their litters (12 males and 10 females) and additionally, one male and six females. These animals were obtained from the Cancer Research Laboratories, University of Birmingham, where by brother × sister mating they had been maintained through 21 generations. The Birmingham C57BL strain was originally obtained in 1950 from the Department of Experimental Pathology and Cancer Research, University of Leeds. Since 1959, the Colworth colony has been maintained as an inbred strain by brother × sister mating. Breeding stock are maintained in metal "shoe-box" cages with absorbent wood shavings as litter and nesting material. Stock pelleted diet and water are available *ad lib*. Average litter size is 6.1 and both males and females are weaned at 24–25 days (9–10 g). Weanlings are maintained in plastic cages, six or seven of the same sex per cage, and have access to stock pelleted diet *ad lib*. Mice selected for experimental studies are kept under these conditions until at least 6 weeks old and are put on test after they reach 17 g or more body weight.

When animals are introduced to a test, they are transferred to metal cages in an experimental room; each cage is composed of five cells in which animals are housed individually. The diet fed to experimental mice is dependent on the treatment employed. On long-term studies (80–100 weeks) of the effects of cutaneous application, subcutaneous injection or administration of the test compound in drinking water, stock pelleted diet is fed. On long-term feeding studies, however, a semi-synthetic purified (SSP) diet is usually employed, particularly when inclusion of the test compound is at a level higher than 1·0% of the diet. SSP diets are fed freshly to mice twice weekly; food intake and weekly weight of each mouse are recorded.

In practice, when SSP diet is used as a vehicle for test compounds in long-term feeding studies, it is usual to include a control group fed stock pelleted diet, as well as a control group fed SSP diet. A positive carcinogen control group is also often included, the nature of the carcinogen being dependent upon the type of study being undertaken *e.g.* cutaneous application, feeding, *etc.* In studies of food additives containing appreciable quantities of mineral salts, *e.g.* sodium chloride, additional control groups may be included, the SSP diet fed to these groups containing levels of mineral salts equivalent to those in the test diets containing the food additive. In long-term studies, 40 male and 40 female mice are usually started in each group.

All animals are inspected daily and signs of ill health or reaction to treatment recorded. All mice dying or killed during the trials or at their termination are submitted to post-mortem examination and at necropsy, all macroscopic abnormalities are recorded. Except in cases of advanced autolysis, portions of all major organs are retained for histological examination. At necropsy, the number, size, location and appearance of each nodule in the liver is recorded; after weighing the organ, multiple sections are made through each lobe and portions of each lobe exhibiting focal macroscopic lesions are retained for histological examination. In the absence of significant macroscopic pathology, paraffin blocks are prepared routinely from the left, median and right anterior lobes, while frozen sections, stained by the Oil Red O method, are prepared from the median lobe. The histological features of each nodule and of the surrounding hepatic parenchyma are recorded.

DIET

Stock pelleted diet used in this laboratory is manufactured by our own Company from natural ingredients. It provides for normal growth, reproduction and maintenance of laboratory rats and mice. Since it is composed of natural ingredients, variations in nutrient quality between batches may be expected. Contamination with herbicide or insecticide residues or toxic microbial products formed during storage may occur. The SSP diet is baked and fed in biscuit form.

The composition and chemical analysis of the two diets is given in Tables I, II and III. Stock pelleted diet contains more of all the nutrients per unit of weight with the exception of oil, sodium and energy. These analyses, however, fail to take account of the digestibility of nutrients. The available energy from stock diet and purified diet is 2·84 and 4·13 cal/g respectively in the rat.

A further point of interest is the larger size of the intestine and its contents in

TABLE I

COMPOSITION OF DIETS

Stock pelleted diet (%)		Semi synthetic purified diet (SSP) (%)	
Wheatfeed	25·94	White wheat flour	50·0
Buttermilk	12·56	Casein	20·0
Groundnut meal (extracted)	10·09	Groundnut oil	10·0
Maize	10·09	Cellulose powder	6·0
Coconut meal (expelled)	10·09	Vitamin B supplement[a]	6·0
White fish meal	8·40	Jones–Foster salt mix[a]	4·0
Dried yeast	8·00	Liver extract	1·0
Molasses	5·04	Folic acid in starch[a]	1·0
Barley	5·04	p-Aminobenzoic acid in starch[a]	1·0
Wheat germ	2·52	Wheat germ oil	1·0
Salt	1·00		
Compound colour	0·84		
Lime	0·33		
Mineral mix	0·06		
Vitamin mix	+		

(1) An oral supplement of 50 I.U. Vitamin A and 5 I.U. Vitamin D is given in groundnut oil once weekly.
(2) When a lower level of groundnut oil is included in SSP diet, the level of white wheat flour is proportionately increased.

[a] Composition in Table II.

TABLE II

SSP DIET-SPECIFIC INGREDIENT COMPOSITION

(1) Jones–Foster salt mix (g)		
Potassium phosphate	KH_2PO_4	3266.0
Calcium carbonate	$CaCO_3$ heavy	3204.0
Sodium chloride	NaCl recrystallised	1170.0
Magnesium sulphate	$MgSO_4$ dried	482.0
Ferrous sulphate	$FeSO_4.7H_2O$	226.0
Manganese sulphate	$MnSO_4.4H_2O$	44.60
Potassium iodide	KI	6.64
Copper sulphate	$CuSO_4.5H_2O$	4.00
Zinc chloride	$ZnCl_2$	2.18
Cobalt chloride	$CoCl_2.6H_2O$	0.20
(2) Vitamin B supplement (g)		
Choline chloride		80.00
Nicotinic acid (Niacin)		12.00
Pantothenic acid		0.60
Riboflavin		0.13
Ascorbic acid		0.10
Thiamine hydrochloride (Aneurine)		0.10
Pyridoxine		0.06
Starch		1000.00
(3) Folic acid in starch (g)		
Folic acid		15.00
Starch		985.00
(4) p-Aminobenzoic acid in starch (g)		
p-Aminobenzoic acid		100.00
Starch		900.00

TABLE III

CHEMICAL ANALYSES OF DIETS

Analysis given is for SSP diet containing 10% groundnut oil.

	Stock pelleted diet	SSP
Moisture %	10·0	8·1
Protein %	26·3	22·7
Fat %	4·5	11·3
Fibre %	4·9	3·3
Ash %	6·8	3·7
Energy (Cal/g)	4·15	4·78

animals fed stock diet. In any consideration of body weight, it must be appreciated that, because a much higher proportion of the body weight of animals fed stock diet is intestine and contents, the carcase weight of these animals is much reduced when compared to animals fed SSP diet.

In most of our studies, mice have been fed SSP diet containing 10.0% groundnut oil (total dietary fat 11.3%) but in a smaller series, only 4.0–5.0% groundnut oil was included in the SSP diets (total dietary fat 4.8–6.3%). In this paper, for convenience, mice fed 11·3% fat in SSP diet will be referred to as the *10·0% groundnut oil group* while the groups fed 4·8–6·3% fat will be referred to as the *5·0% groundnut oil group*. In order to achieve uniformity in interpretation, only those studies in which histological examination has been undertaken by the author will be included.

PATHOLOGY

Macroscopic

At necropsy of mice killed at the end of 80-week studies, striking differences are observed in the appearance of the liver, depending on the diet fed. In mice fed stock pelleted diet, the organ is usually normal in outline and pale brown in colour; in contrast, the livers of mice fed SSP diet are frequently yellow/golden in colour and greasy in consistency with rounded edges. Mice fed SSP diet are obese. Animals fed stock diet, on the other hand, are seldom obese. The only other significant macroscopic difference observed between mice fed the two diets concerns the degree of enlargement of the accessory sex glands. Over 85% of male mice fed SSP diet show gross enlargement of the vesicular glands; in a recent study the mean weight of the glands in mice fed SSP diet was 5·9 g representing 13·6% of terminal body weight. In contrast, gross vesicular gland enlargement is much less common in mice fed stock pelleted diet and in its severe form is identified in only approximately 18% of male animals.

The livers of Colworth C57BL mice frequently show a variety of lesions at necropsy and differentiation of proliferative parenchymal foci may be difficult. Hepatic haemangiomata are frequently bright red/purple in colour and unlike focal parenchymal nodules, are not sharply demarcated from adjacent parenchyma.

Parenchymal nodules are usually circular or oval in shape and may be elevated above the hepatic surface but in some locations, particularly on the diaphragmatic surface, they may assume a flattened plaque formation. Some large superficial nodules may be pedunculated, attached to the liver by a thin strand of atrophic hepatic tissue. Occasionally, these nodules may become grossly enlarged due to vascular engorgement as a sequel to torsion. Livers containing nodules never show macroscopic evidence of cirrhosis.

Parenchymal nodules vary in size from 1–30 mm in diameter and may be single or multiple, the maximum number identified in any one liver in this series being eleven. Small nodules (1–4 mm) are uniformly yellow or brown, sharply demarcated and softer and more homogeneous in consistency than the surrounding parenchyma. A small proportion of these nodules are distinctly white in colour and glossy in appearance. Larger nodules (4–10 mm) seldom show the uniformity of structure and colour observed in smaller lesions. Frequently, they are mottled yellow, brown and red, and over the surface of some, a clearly defined network of thin-walled blood vessels may be visible. The cut surface of such nodules is occasionally highly vascular and of very soft consistency. Nodules over 10 mm diameter resemble the 4–10 mm series but in the former, a rich superficial vascular network is a consistent feature. Many of the largest nodules have a central, superficial crater associated with necrosis within the nodule while some are multilobulate. Although the majority of large nodules are covered by a smooth capsule, a few show superficial fibrinous adhesions to adjacent viscera and are readily ruptured *in vivo* and at necropsy.

Although approximately 80% of all nodules are visible on the surface, the remainder occur deep in the hepatic substance. This deeper location is more frequently noted towards the diaphragmatic surface of the left and median lobes and may be detected only on multiple section of the organ. This must be considered when counting nodules. Despite the presence of large nodules in close proximity to the gall bladder and major intrahepatic bile ducts, icterus has been identified in only a few mice, all fed known hepatocarcinogens. In these cases, multiple large nodules were present throughout the liver. Likewise, ascites has seldom been observed except in mice fed the hepato-carcinogen butter yellow.

Macroscopic pulmonary metastases from primary hepatic neoplasms are extremely rare in untreated Colworth C57BL mice, only five such instances having been confirmed histologically during the present studies. In each of these cases, multiple nodules up to 2 mm diameter were identified in all lobes of the lung.

HISTOPATHOLOGY

(a) "Normal" liver

There are striking differences in the histology of the livers of mice fed stock pelleted diet or SSP diet for 80 weeks, the most significant being the amount of neutral fat present in parenchymal cells. In mice fed stock diet, parenchymal cell lipid is mainly centrilobular in distribution while the presence of neutral fat in Kupffer cells is frequently seen. In contrast, the feeding of SSP diet results in massive accumulation of intracytoplasmic parenchymal lipid in all zones of all hepatic lobules (Figs. 1 and 2). In many animals, tiny droplets or larger globules of neutral fat are identified in a proportion of parenchymal nuclei. Diffuse fibrosis is not a feature of either group, while adenofibrosis (cholangiofibrosis) is observed with approximately equal but low frequency in both.

A wide variety of other lesions is consistently identified in the livers of ageing Colworth C57BL mice. These include nuclear enlargement and binucleate paren-chymal cells, periportal lymphocytic infiltration and focal necrosis of single cells or small clusters of hepatocytes. Neither the incidence nor the intensity of these features is influenced by the diets used.

Several other changes differ in frequency depending upon the diet, being more common in mice fed SSP diet. These changes include centrilobular hypertrophy, multinucleate hepatocytes (Fig. 4), nuclei with condensed chromatin (Fig. 5) and

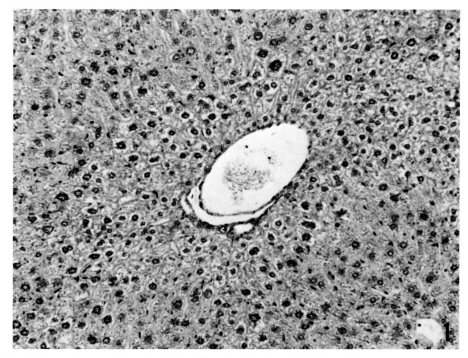

Fig. 1. Liver of mouse fed stock diet for 80 weeks. Lendrum's M.S.B. × 180.

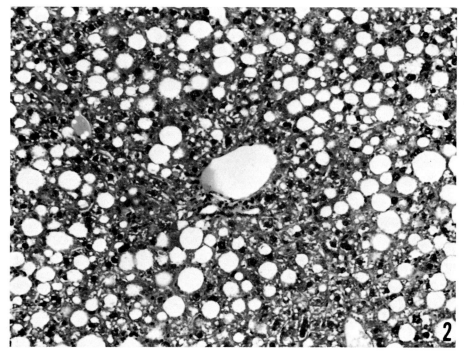

Fig. 2. Extensive accumulation of neutral fat in liver of mouse fed SSP diet (10·0% groundnut oil) for 80 weeks. H.P.S. × 180.

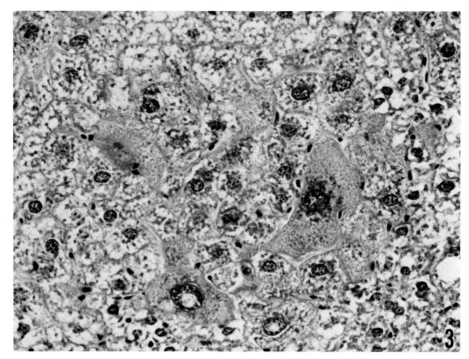

Fig. 3. Cytoplasmic and nuclear enlargement (focal hypertrophy) in liver of mouse fed SSP diet (5·0% groundnut oil) for 80 weeks. Lendrum's M.S.B. × 335.

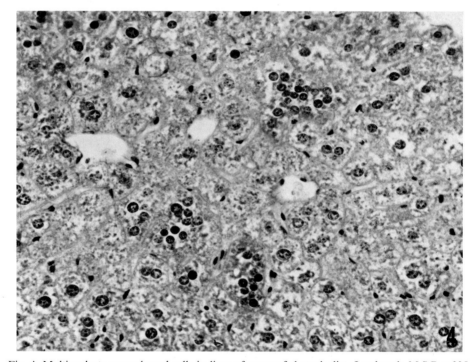

Fig. 4. Multinucleate parenchymal cells in liver of mouse fed stock diet. Lendrum's M.S.B. × 335.

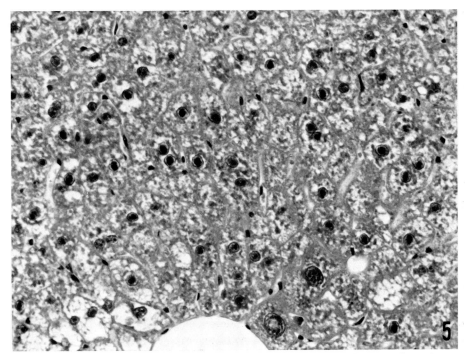

Fig. 5. Condensation of parenchymal nuclear chromatin in periphery of left lobe liver of mouse fed SSP diet (5·0% groundnut oil) H.P.S. × 335.

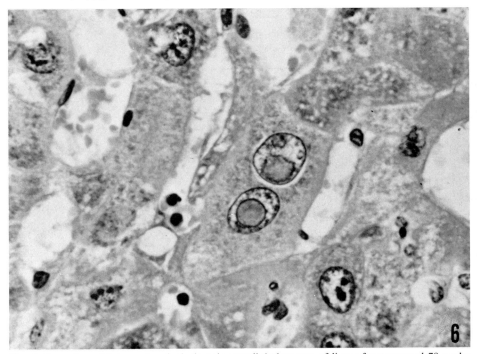

Fig. 6. Parenchymal intranuclear inclusions in centrilobular zone of liver of mouse aged 78 weeks. H.P.S. × 570.

intranuclear inclusions (Fig. 6). Multinucleate parenchymal cells with up to 20 nuclei have been observed in over 65% of mice fed SSP diet and in less than 20% fed stock diet. This feature is identified in all areas of the liver. In contrast, chromatin condensation is observed almost exclusively in the thin peripheral portions of the major hepatic lobes where up to 70% of parenchymal nuclei may be affected.

(b) Focal hypertrophy

Small foci of parenchymal hypertrophy may be observed in animals fed SSP diet. These lesions are composed of clusters of greatly enlarged parenchymal cells (Fig. 3). The cytoplasm of these cells is homogeneous, acidophil and virtually devoid of fat. The nuclei are large and often contain acidophil inclusions. In mice fed stock diet these lesions are rare.

(c) Hepatic parenchymal nodules

Classification

The histological characteristics of any large series of hepatic nodules in Colworth C57BL mice are so numerous and variable in frequency of occurrence and intensity that their classification into distinct categories is fraught with difficulty. However, our classification, in general, agrees with that described in Chapter 3 with an additional separation of the Type A nodules into two categories. The characteristic features of the nodules observed in our studies are listed in Table IV.

TABLE IV

CLASSIFICATION OF HEPATIC PARENCHYMAL NODULES: SUMMARY OF MAIN FEATURES
OF HISTOLOGICAL TYPES[a]

Features	Type 1	Type 2	Type 3
Differentiation	High	Moderate–high	Moderate-poor
Uniformity of cell size	High	Variable	Variable
Cytoplasmic staining affinity	Acidophil	Variable–weakly acidophil to intensely basophil	Basophil
Trabecular development	Poor	Moderate/variable	Well defined
Cytoplasmic lipid	Low	Often high	Low-moderate
Cytoplasmic glycogen	Moderate	Variable	Low
Peripheral compression	Absent	Good	Good
Intravenous permeation	Absent	Rare	Common
Nuclear size	Moderate–large	Variable	Large
Cell size	Large	Variable	Large
Sinusoidal engorgement	Absent	Mild–moderate	Intense
Mitoses	Rare	Variable	Numerous
Intracytoplasmic inclusions	Rare	Common	Rare
Transplantability	Nil	Variable	Frequent

[a] Nodules of Types 1 and 2 are similar to Type A lesions as described by WALKER et al. (1973) and THORPE AND WALKER (1973); Type 3 nodules are equivalent to the Type B lesions described by the same authors.

The first step in this classification was a study of the small number of hepatic nodules which produced pulmonary metastases. Subsequently, all nodules exhibiting the histological characteristics of these malignant neoplasms were designated "Type 3" (hepatocellular carcinomata), irrespective of whether metastases had developed or not. This classification corresponds to the Type B lesion of WALKER et al. (1973). The remaining nodules (Types 1 and 2) constitute Type A of the classification of WALKER et al. (1973). Since a histological description of the lesions has already been presented (Chapter 3), only a summary of the main histological features of the nodules in this series is given (Table IV).

Summary

It is our belief that the hepatic nodules discussed in this communication represent a broad spectrum of pathological change with one feature in common, *viz.* the formation of focal parenchymal lesions. At one end of this spectrum are small foci of hypertrophy/hyperplasia and at the other, malignant neoplasms. Ideally, a classification system of such lesions should take account of both structure and behaviour but since our knowledge of the latter is limited, the system used is based almost exclusively on morphology. The deficiencies of such a system are obvious. Nevertheless, on the basis of observed behaviour and transplantability, it is believed that Type 1 nodules represent foci of hypertrophy and nodular hyperplasia while Type 3 lesions are malignant neoplasms (hepatocellular carcinomata). Type 2 nodules are a mixed group presenting features which suggest a progression from Type 1 but which do not include evidence of malignant transformation.

RESULTS

Effects of diets on nodule incidence, size, distribution and type in untreated mice

Incidence of nodules

The incidence of nodules and multiple nodule formation is higher in mice fed SSP diets than in those receiving stock diet (Table V). The inclusion of 10% groundnut oil in SSP diet results in a greater increase in incidence, particularly in females, than does the feeding of SSP diet containing 5% groundnut oil. On only one occasion did the feeding of SSP diet containing 10% groundnut oil fail to produce an incidence of nodules greater than in animals fed stock diet. The effect of intercurrent disease on nodule incidence in that study (Trial 1) is discussed later.

Size of nodules

The results are summarized in Table VI. It can be seen that nodules in animals fed stock pelleted diet are larger than those in animals fed SSP diets. There is an increased number of nodules on SSP diet which are, however, smaller than those on stock pelleted diet.

TABLE V

EFFECT OF DIET ON ANIMAL SURVIVAL AND INCIDENCE OF MACROSCOPIC AND HISTOLOGICAL HEPATIC PARENCHYMAL NODULES IN UNTREATED MICE AT END OF 80-WEEK STUDIES

Diet	Initial number of mice		Survivors at end of 80-week studies		Percentage survivors		Percentage survivors with nodules		Percentage survivors with single nodules		Percentage survivors with multiple nodules		Total number of nodules		Nodules per survivor	
	M	F	M	F	M	F	M	F	M	F	M	F	M	F	M	F
Macroscopic																
Stock pelleted diet	300	300	276	260	92	87	12	13	10	12	2	1	39	37	0.141	0.142
SSP diet (5.0% groundnut oil)	80	80	64	74	80	93	30	30	25	14	5	16	22	44	0.344	0.595
SSP diet (10.0% groundnut oil)	150	150	101	121	67	81	39	64	28	27	11	36	54	177	0.535	1.463
Histological																
Stock pelleted diet	205	205	184	175	90	85	13	14[a]	11	13	2	1	20	20	0.109	0.114
SSP diet (5.0% groundnut oil)	80	80	64	74	80	93	31	38[a]	25	18	6	20	21	51	0.328	0.689
SSP diet (10.0% groundnut oil)	105	105	70	82	67	78	50	66[a]	37	27	13	39	42	109	0.600	1.329
Histological—Trial 1																
Stock pelleted diet	25	25	13	16	52	64	23	6	23	6			3	1	0.231	0.063
SSP diet (10.0% groundnut oil)	25	25	16	15	64	60	13	13	13	13			2	2	0.125	0.133

[a] Includes nodules identified macroscopically but not present in histological sections.

M, male; F, female.

TABLE VI

EFFECT OF DIET ON SIZE OF HEPATIC PARENCHYMAL NODULES IN UNTREATED MICE AT END OF 80-WEEK STUDIES

Diet	Sex	Percentage survivors with macroscopic nodules	Percentage macroscopic nodules of diameter				Mean macroscopic diameter (mm) of nodules	Mean histological diameter (mm) of nodules
			1–2 mm	3–4 mm	5–9 mm	10 < mm		
Stock pelleted diet	M	12	26	23	28	23	5.64	4.86
	F	13	33	34	19	14	4.94	4.29
	M and F	13	29	29	24	18	5.30	4.58
SSP diet (5.0% groundnut oil)	M	30	32	27	14	27	5.15	4.27
	F	30	59	30	9	2	2.87	1.82
	M and F	30	49	29	11	11	3.63	2.53
SSP diet (10.0% groundnut oil)	M	39	42	28	19	11	3.44	2.40
	F	64	44	32	13	11	3.30	2.92
	M and F	52	44	31	14	11	3.33	2.77

TABLE VII

LOBAR DISTRIBUTION OF HEPATIC PARENCHYMAL NODULES IN UNTREATED MICE AT END OF 80-WEEK STUDIES

Diet	Sex	Total nodules (site recorded)	Left lobe		Median lobe		Right lobe	
			Number of nodules	Percentage of total nodules	Number of nodules	Percentage of total nodules	Number of nodules	Percentage of total nodules
Stock pelleted diet	M	36	17	47	10	28	9	25
	F	35	10	29	12	34	13	37
	M and F	71	27	38	22	31	22	31
SSP diet (5.0% groundnut oil)	M	20	7	35	7	35	6	30
	F	37	9	24	15	41	13	35
	M and F	57	16	28	22	39	19	33
SSP diet (10% groundnut oil)	M	54	17	31	26	48	11	21
	F	174	43	25	61	35	70	40
	M and F	228	60	26	87	38	81	36

TABLE VIII

EFFECT OF DIET ON THE INCIDENCE OF NODULES OF DIFFERENT HISTOLOGICAL TYPES IDENTIFIED IN UNTREATED MICE AT END OF 80-WEEK STUDIES

Diet	Sex	Number of surviving mice	Number of histological nodules	Percentage of nodules diagnosed as				Percentage survivors with nodules of			
				Focal hyper-trophy	Type 1	Type 2	Type 3	Focal hyper-trophy	Type 1	Type 2	Type 3
Stock pelleted diet	M	184	20		50	25	25		4	3	3
	F	175	20		45	35	20		5	4	2
	M and F	359	40		48	30	23		5	4	3
SSP diet (5.0% groundnut oil)	M	64	21	5	57	29	10	2	16	8	3
	F	74	51	8	68	22	2	4	28	7	1
	M and F	138	72	7	65	24	4	3	23	7	2
SSP diet (10.0% groundnut oil)	M	70	42	7	64	27	2	3	33	16	1
	F	82	109	9	45	39	7	8	38	34	9
	M and F	152	151	8	51	35	6	7	36	26	5

TABLE IX

EFFECT OF DIET AND INTERCURRENT DISEASE ON BODY WEIGHT GAIN, FOOD CONSUMPTION AND FOOD CONVERSION OF UNTREATED MICE DURING 80-WEEK STUDIES

Diet	Sex	Initial body weight (g)	Body weight (g) at 80 weeks	Body weight gain (g)	Food consumption (g)	Food conversion[a]	Body weight gain (g) between weeks					
							0–6	7–12	13–20	21–40	41–60	61–80
Stock pelleted diet	M	21.1	37.4	16.3	—	—	4.0	2.5	2.2	4.1	2.7	0.8
	F	17.2	34.5	17.3	—	—	3.5	2.1	2.2	4.8	3.9	0.8
SSP diet (5.0% groundnut oil)	M	20.1	42.7	22.6	1839	0.0123	5.1	2.8	2.6	5.3	4.6	2.2
	F	16.7	41.5	24.8	1858	0.0133	4.5	1.5	2.6	6.0	6.0	4.2
SSP diet (10% groundnut oil)	M	21.3	44.6	23.3	1841	0.0127	4.9	3.4	3.3	6.2	3.3	2.2
	F	18.0	45.9	27.9	1876	0.0148	4.2	3.7	3.5	7.5	5.4	3.6
Trial 1												
Stock pelleted diet	M	21.3	32.7	11.4	—	—	4.2	1.1	2.3	1.5	1.0	1.3
	F	16.7	31.2	14.5	—	—	3.9	1.4	1.9	2.5	3.1	1.7
SSP diet (10% groundnut oil)	M	21.9	35.2	13.3	1806	0.0074	3.5	1.5	2.6	1.7	3.4	0.6
	F	17.1	39.2	22.1	1760	0.0126	3.7	1.5	3.2	3.9	6.9	2.9

[a] Food conversion: Body weight gain (g)/food intake (g).

TABLE X

EFFECT OF DIET AND INTERCURRENT DISEASE ON BODY WEIGHT GAIN, TERMINAL BODY WEIGHT AND ORGAN WEIGHTS OF UNTREATED MICE ON 80-WEEK STUDIES

Diet	Sex	Weeks taken to attain body weight of				Terminal body weight (g)[a]	Liver weight		Kidneys weight		Testes weight	
		25 g	30 g	35 g	40 g		Absolute (g)	Relative	Absolute (g)	Relative	Absolute (g)	Relative
Stock pelleted diet	M	6.3	20.8	45.5	NA[b]	37.7	2.13	5.64	0.58	1.54	0.138	0.366
	F	20.0	40.0	80.0	NA	35.2	1.92	5.44	0.54	1.52	—	—
SSP diet (5.0% groundnut oil)	M	5.5	18.0	35.5	57.5	41.1	2.38	5.79	0.49	1.19	0.121	0.292
	F	19.0	37.5	54.5	70.5	40.3	2.39	5.93	0.41	1.02	—	—
SSP diet (10% groundnut oil)	M	4.0	12.0	22.0	38.5	45.0	2.88	6.40	0.57	1.27	0.119	0.261
	F	11.6	21.3	34.8	53.5	45.8	3.43	7.48	0.50	1.09	—	—
Trial 1 Stock pelleted diet	M	5.0	40.0	NA	NA	32.3	1.99	6.16	0.65	2.01	0.171	0.526
	F	28.0	64.0	NA	NA	31.6	1.72	5.44	0.59	1.87	—	—
SSP diet (10% groundnut oil)	M	5.0	28.0	80.0	NA	35.2	2.54	7.22	0.68	1.93	0.179	0.511
	F	18.0	44.0	60.0	NA	39.2	2.26	5.77	0.53	1.35	—	—

[a] Body weight at necropsy (80–82 weeks after commencement of studies).

[b] NA, not attained.

Lobar distribution of nodules

Mice fed stock pelleted diet had nodules equally distributed throughout the three main hepatic lobes (Table VII); in animals fed SSP diets, there was a slight shift in distribution from the left to the median and right lobes.

Type of nodules

The greater number of histological nodules observed in mice fed SSP diets was attributable to the development of foci of hypertrophy and an increase in the number of Types 1 and 2 nodules; the number of Type 3 nodules was not influenced significantly by the feeding of SSP diets. In mice fed SSP diets containing 10% groundnut oil, the percentage survivors with nodules of Type 2 was greater than in animals fed diets containing 5% of the oil (Table VIII); this effect was more marked in females than in males.

Effect of intercurrent disease on nodule formation

The first 80 week mouse feeding study (Trial 1) undertaken in this laboratory was initiated in 1959 and included untreated groups fed stock pelleted diet and purified diet containing SSP 10% groundnut oil diet. Survival in the untreated groups was 60%. The histological incidence of hepatic parenchymal nodules (unspecified) in untreated mice killed at 80 weeks was low − 13·0 and 13·7% respectively in animals fed stock diet and SSP diet (Table V). Comparison of data from Trial 1 with information acquired from later 80-week studies has highlighted several major differences attributable to disease:

(a) Body weight gains and terminal body weights of mice fed SSP diet were much lower than in any comparable subsequent study (Tables IX and X; Figs. 7 and 8).

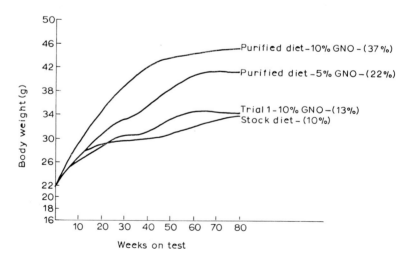

Fig. 7. Body weight gain and terminal incidence of hepatic parenchymal nodules in male mice fed stock diet or SSP diet for 80 weeks. Figures in parentheses indicate % incidence of nodules.

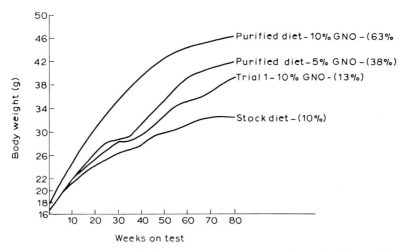

Fig. 8. Body weight gain and terminal incidence of hepatic parenchymal nodules in female mice fed stock diet or SSP diet for 80 weeks. Figures in parentheses indicate % incidence of nodules.

(b) Food conversion in both sexes and absolute and relative hepatic weights in females were lower than in any comparable study (Tables IX and X).

(c) Absolute and relative renal weights were higher than in any other 80-week feeding study (Table X).

(d) Terminal survival was the poorest ever recorded in any 80-week study (Table V). These observations were associated with a high incidence of amyloidosis, mite infestation and cutaneous ulceration.

The role of dietary lipid

Since evidence accumulated over many years has indicated that the incidence of hepatic nodules in Colworth C57BL mice is influenced significantly by the diet fed and by the level of groundnut oil incorporated in SSP diet, recent studies have been directed towards assessment of the role of dietary lipid. Evaluation of a study of 1200 mice fed 6 different diets and killed after 12, 26, 52 and 80 weeks is not yet complete but some preliminary results are available.

While these confirm an association between dietary lipid and hepatic nodule formation they also clearly demonstrate that other factors are involved. Thus while the addition of 10% groundnut oil to *stock diet* substantially increased the frequency with which nodules were observed, the incidence recorded was much lower than that associated with the inclusion of 10% groundnut oil in *SSP diet*. Likewise, the feeding of SSP diet without groundnut oil produced an incidence of nodules lower than that associated with inclusion of the oil but still significantly higher than that resulting from the feeding of stock diet (HOPE *et al.*, unpublished observations). It is thus apparent that although dietary lipid is one factor associated with hepatic parenchymal nodule formation in mice, other aspects of the aetiology of this lesion remain unresolved.

Relevant background data

Growth

Mice fed SSP diet grow more rapidly and attain a greater terminal body weight than those fed stock diet; growth and terminal body weight are greater in animals fed SSP 10 % groundnut oil diet than in those fed the 5 % groundnut oil diet (Table IX). Body weight gain of female mice fed 10% groundnut oil in SSP diet is the greatest of either sex fed any of the three diets. Body weight gain of animals fed stock diet is consistently lower than that of mice fed SSP diet but performance on stock diet is particularly poor between weeks 61 and 80 (Table IX). When a comparison is made of the number of weeks taken for mice to attain body weights of 25, 30, 35 and 40 g (Table X), the differences are striking. Neither male nor female animals fed stock diet attain group means of 40 g; indeed, females fed this diet only just reach 35 g before necropsy at 80 weeks. In contrast, mice fed SSP diet reach a mean body weight of 40 g after 38·5–70·5 weeks, males fed SSP 10% groundnut oil diet attaining this weight most rapidly.

Comparison of rate of growth, terminal body weight and incidence of hepatic parenchymal nodules reveals an interesting correlation. Rapid growth and high terminal body weight are associated with a high incidence of nodules while a similar correlation exists between slower growth, lower terminal body weight and a low incidence of nodules.

Food consumption (Table IX)

Due to the crumbly nature of pellets of stock diet and the loss of considerable quantities of this diet in the bedding, estimation of consumption of stock diet is not accurate. The food consumption of mice fed SSP diets containing 5·0 and 10% groundnut oil is very similar during 80-week feeding trials. Food utilisation (body weight gain (g)/food intake (g)) is slightly better in mice fed 10% groundnut oil in SSP diet.

Organ weights (Table X)

The absolute and relative weights of the liver are greater in mice fed SSP diet than in those fed stock diet, the effect of 10% groundnut oil in SSP diet producing a marked increase in both absolute and relative hepatic weights of female mice. There is a close relationship between hepatic weight and the incidence of nodules in this organ, best exemplified by the similarity of weight and incidence of nodules in both sexes fed SSP 5% groundnut oil diet and the greater hepatic weight and higher incidence of nodules in females fed the SSP 10% groundnut oil diet.

EFFECTS OF TREATMENT

Carcinogens (Tables XI and XII)

The susceptibility of the Colworth C57BL mouse to known carcinogens has been

TABLE XI

EFFECTS OF THE INCLUSION IN SSP DIETS OF A KNOWN CARCINOGEN, SODIUM CHLORIDE AND TWO FOOD ADDITIVES ON THE INCIDENCE OF HEPATIC PARENCHYMAL NODULES IN MICE AT THE END OF 80-WEEK FEEDING STUDIES

Diet/additive	Initial number of mice		Percentage survivors		Percentage survivors with nodules		Percentage survivors with single nodule		Percentage survivors with multiple nodules		Total number of macroscopic nodules		Macroscopic nodules per survivor	
	M	F	M	F	M	F	M	F	M	F	M	F	M	F
Known hepatocarcinogen														
SSP diet + 0.06% Butter Yellow[b]	30	30	60	37	100	100			100	100	a		a	
Food additive—Flavour G														
SSP diet (10.0% groundnut oil)	90	90	69	80	37	63	26	26	11	37	33	110	0.532	1.527
SSP diet + NaCl = 5.0% additive[b,d]	90	90	68	76	39	75	28	28	11	47	36	133	0.590	1.953
SSP diet + NaCl = 9.0% additive[b]	90	90	79	80	32	69	18	26	14	43	41	118	0.577	1.638
SSP diet + 5.0% additive[b]	90	90	74	80	45	89	19	17	26	72	54	217	0.805	3.013
SSP diet + 9.0% additive[b]	90	90	81	84	42	86	16	20	26	66	64	222	0.876	2.921
Food additive—Colour F														
SSP diet (5.0% groundnut oil)[c]	40	40	80	93	38	22	31	14	7	8	14	17	0.437	0.459
SSP diet + 0.0125% additive[c]	40	40	93	90	25	28	22	11	3	17	10	20	0.270	0.555
SSP diet + 0.0375% additive[c]	40	40	97	80	16	44	16	6		38	6	40	0.153	1.250
SSP diet + 0.075% additive[c]	40	40	90	95	45	53	33	24	12	29	20	48	0.555	1.263
SSP diet + 0.125% additive[c]	40	40	100	93	33	54	28	19	5	35	15	51	0.375	1.378

a At necropsy, nodules were too numerous and too closely apposed to count or measure satisfactorily.
b SSP diet containing 10.0% groundnut oil.
c SSP diet containing 5.0% groundnut oil.
d In one group of 45 female mice fed SSP diet with added sodium chloride, a nodule incidence of 87% was recorded.

TABLE XII

EFFECTS OF THE INCLUSION, IN SSP DIETS, OF A KNOWN CARCINOGEN, SODIUM CHLORIDE AND TWO FOOD ADDITIVES ON THE INCIDENCE OF HEPATIC PARENCHYMAL NODULES OF DIFFERENT HISTOLOGICAL TYPES IN MICE AT THE END OF 80-WEEK TRIALS

Diet/additive	Percentage of total nodules diagnosed as								Percentage of survivors with nodules diagnosed as							
	Focal hypertrophy		Type 1		Type 2		Type 3		Focal hypertrophy		Type 1		Type 2		Type 3	
	M	F	M	F	M	F	M	F	M	F	M	F	M	F	M	F
Known carcinogen																
SSP diet + 0.06% Butter Yellow[b]	a	a	a	a	a	a	a	a	100	100	100	100	100	100	67	91
Food additive—Flavour G																
SSP diet (10% groundnut oil)	6	8	64	49	23	33	7	10	3	7	31	36	13	27	3	12
SSP diet + NaCl = 5.0% additive[b,d]	6	9	57	44	27	30	10	17	3	13	36	41	21	37	11	8
SSP diet + NaCl = 9.0% additive[b]	7	7	53	51	21	37	19	5	3	8	27	40	15	27	12	6
SSP diet + 5.0% additive[b]	3	6	76	63	17	25	4	6	4	14	33	63	21	36	3	11
SSP diet + 9.0% additive[b]	6	8	63	65	15	22	16	5	3	10	30	68	18	43	6	14
Food additive—Colour F																
SSP diet (5.0% groundnut oil)	7		50	63	29	37	14		3		25	20	6	9	3	3
SSP diet + 0.0125% additive[c]		5	67	70	19	25	14			3	19	20	7	6	3	3
SSP diet + 0.0375% additive[c]		3	74	67	16	25	10	5		3	16	34	5	9	3	3
SSP diet + 0.075% additive[c]	5	4	75	83	15	8	5	5	3	5	36	45	6	11	3	3
SSP diet + 0.125% additive[c]	6	2	79	87	11	7	4		3	3	28	43	8	11	3	3

a At necropsy, nodules were too numerous and too closely apposed to count satisfactorily.

b SSP diet containing 10.0% groundnut oil.

c SSP diet containing 5.0% groundnut oil.

d In one group of 45 female mice fed SSP diet with added sodium chloride, a nodule incidence of 87% was recorded.

demonstrated by its response to the cutaneous application of 9,10-dimethyl-1,2-benz-anthracene (DMBA) (PHILP, 1963), and to the intubation of 3,4-benzpyrene and 20-methylcholanthrene. None of these carcinogens significantly influenced the incidence of hepatic neoplasia but 4-dimethylaminoazobenzene (butter yellow) proved to be a potent hepatocarcinogen when fed at a 0·06 % level in SSP diet. This resulted in heavy mortality (51·8 %) before the end of an 80-week trial. Of 31 deaths, 22 were attributed to the development of Type 3 nodules (hepatocellular carcinoma) with severe anaemia and/or gross ascites; 16 of these cases were females and 6 males.

The first death attributable to a malignant hepatic tumour occurred during week 47 of the study. Of the 29 animals fed the carcinogen and surviving to the end of the study, 23 (79 %) had developed multiple hepatocellular carcinomata; 13 were males and 10 females. Multiple nodules of Types 1 and 2 were identified in all surviving mice. Pulmonary metastases from Type 3 nodules were present in only 3 animals, 2 of which were females. The most striking features of this study were the high proportion of animals which developed Type 3 nodules (hepatocellular carcinoma) and the presence of multiple parenchymal nodules, predominantly of Type 2, in all mice surviving to the end of the 80-week trial.

Food additives (Tables XI and XII)

Three food additives studied in this laboratory increased the incidence of hepatic parenchymal nodule formation. Since two of the three are closely related chemically and since the results for both are similar, they will be considered together (Flavour G); the third (Food Colour F) will be considered separately.

Flavour G was fed to mice at dietary levels of 5·0 and 9·0 % in SSP diet containing 10 % groundnut oil; since the sodium chloride content of the flavour was high (approx. 23 %), control groups fed similar levels of sodium chloride only were included in this study. Survival was not adversely affected by feeding the flavour but the number of survivors with macroscopic parenchymal nodules was greater in both flavour groups than in control animals fed SSP diet with or without added salt. On histological examination, no increase in the proportion of nodules diagnosed as Type 3 or in the percentage survivors with nodules of this Type was observed. The percentage of survivors with nodules of Type 1 was increased, particularly in females (Table XII). No dose response was noted. It is concluded that the increased incidence of hepatic parenchymal nodules observed in mice fed additive flavour G was not due to an increased incidence of Type 3 (hepatocellular carcinoma) but was due mainly to an increased occurrence of Type 1 nodules (nodular hyperplasia).

Food colour F was incorporated in SSP diet containing the lower dietary level (5 %) of groundnut oil. Survival was not adversely affected by inclusion of the colour but the incidence of hepatic nodules in female mice fed the higher levels of the additive was at least twice as high as that observed in untreated animals. No effect on nodule incidence was noted in mice fed the lowest dietary level of the food colour. As in the case of Flavour G, the increased incidence of nodules was mainly attributable to an increase in Type 1; the frequency of occurrence of Type 3 (hepatocellular carcinoma) was not influenced. Again, however, no clearly defined dose response was associated with the feeding of the additive.

In both, it has been shown that the additional nodules observed are predominantly small in size and of histological Type 1; no increase in hepatocellular carcinoma has been demonstrated. These effects are very similar to those produced by dietary change from stock diet to SSP diet containing 10% groundnut oil.

DISCUSSION

The influence of the degree of calorie restriction on the formation of a number of tumours has been studied. For several tumours, including the spontaneous hepatoma of mice (TANNENBAUM AND SILVERSTONE, 1949), the magnitude of tumour inhibition is dependent on the degree of restriction. Moreover, decrease in the mean size of hepatomas with decrease in calorie intake suggests that the hepatic tumours may have originated later in the more restricted groups. As pointed out by TANNENBAUM AND SILVERSTONE (1949), however, statistical evaluation of the results of calorie restriction on hepatoma formation indicate that the point of maximum change in tumour incidence is not dependent on a particular level of calorie intake but rather, is determined by the range of incidences between the highest and lowest levels of food intake. The largest inhibition of hepatoma formation for proportionate reduction in food intake, occurs near the level of 50% tumour incidence. As might be expected, however, a sufficiently potent carcinogenic stimulus can overcome the effect of calorie restriction, although an increase in tumour latency may still be detectable (TANNENBAUM, 1945).

These classical studies from TANNENBAUM's laboratory obviously focus attention on the mechanism of action of calorie restriction in relation to reduced tumour incidence; to date, there is no satisfactory explanation of this effect. Initially, it was considered by TANNENBAUM (1942) that the effect of calorie restriction was a general one, insofar as it affects the relative weights of organs, constituents of tissues and body fluids, hormone levels, metabolism, etc. Subsequently, however, attention was focused on an interaction between calorie restriction and the endocrine system. This concept was based on the hypothesis that the reduced incidence of spontaneous mammary tumours, observed in mice following dietary restriction (TANNENBAUM, 1940; 1947), was due principally to a diminished production of oestrogen, assumed to be the primary carcinogen (HUSEBY et al., 1945). Thereafter, the greater susceptibility of male mice to spontaneous hepatoma formation reported by numerous authors, including BURNS AND SCHENKEN (1940), GORER (1940), LIPPINCOTT et al. (1942), MILLER AND PYBUS (1945), ANDERVONT (1950), AGNEW AND GARDNER (1952) and HESTON AND VLAHAKIS (1966) suggested that a hormonal factor could be associated with the development of hepatic parenchymal tumours. The observation by HESTON (1963) that the occurrence of spontaneous hepatomas in highly susceptible (C3H × YBR)F$_1$ male mice was completely inhibited by hypophysectomy appeared to support the hormonal hypothesis. However, the recent report by ROWLATT et al. (1973) that the same result can be achieved, in the same strain, by dietary restriction must once again raise doubts concerning the importance of an endocrine interaction with dietary restriction.

While great attention is rightly paid to the work of TANNENBAUM and his associates concerning the effects of calorie restriction on tumour formation, several other highly significant observations on the relationship between diet and the incidence of hepatomas in mice have been reported. The earliest was that of STRONG (1938) who observed a slight increase in the incidence of hepatomas in CBA mice when the diet fed was changed from one of rolled oats, meat scrap, powdered whole milk and salt (oatmeal diet) to a commercial one (Purina fox chow). At the same time, it was noted that the animals lived longer on the commercial diet and since the CBA strain had been developed for longevity, a higher incidence of spontaneous tumours was expected. In this early work the inadequacies of available diets are only apparent if the publications are closely studied. Thus, BURNS AND SCHENKEN (1940) report that lettuce was given to breeding stock when breeding performance was poor, while Gorer (1940) added a seed mixture to a commercially available diet.

In a study of spontaneous hepatomas in mice of strains C3H and CBA, ANDERVONT (1950), obviously considered that some of the differences in the incidence of hepatoma formation observed in C3H mice may have been due to the feeding of different diets (Purina dog chow and Purina laboratory chow). Subsequently, in a short communication, SILVERSTONE et al. (1952) reported that the incidence of spontaneous hepatomas was considerably higher in DBA and C3H mice fed diets, composed of casein, cornstarch, partially hydrogenated cottonseed oil, synthetic vitamins and a salt mixture, than in mice of the same strains fed commercial diets, composed principally of natural food (Purina laboratory chow, etc.). The authors did not give details of dietary composition or hepatoma incidence.

From 1950 onwards, a series of papers from HESTON's laboratory drew attention to the increasing incidence of hepatomas in strain C3H mice (HESTON et al., 1950; HESTON AND DERINGER, 1952; HESTON AND DERINGER, 1953; DERINGER, 1959) but, by 1959, the highest incidence of hepatomas ever recorded in any strain of mice was reported in strain C3HeB. HESTON et al. (1960) confirmed a very high incidence in males of 3 substrains of strain C3H fed NCI pellets (formerly Derwood pellets) as used by DERINGER (1959). Since much of the earlier data on strain C3H had been obtained from mice fed Purina laboratory chow or Purina dog chow, an additional group of substrain C3Hf was included in this study and fed Purina laboratory chow instead of NCI pellets. In the group fed Purina chow, the incidence of hepatomas was statistically significantly lower than in the group of the same substrain fed NCI pellets. The caloric value and the fat content of the NCI pellets were higher than in the chow, but the protein content lower; growth rate was slightly higher on the NCI pellets.

Support for a dietary role in hepatoma formation was soon forthcoming. Reciprocal hybrids of strains DBA/2WyDi and CE/J had been maintained at the Jackson Laboratory, Bar Harbor, since 1942 and from 1942–58 the incidence of hepatomas in these hybrid males was less than 1 % at 28–32 months. During this period the mice were fed Purina fox chow and Purina laboratory chow ad lib. In 1958, however, a new diet (Old Guilford Diet) conforming to the Morris formula (17–19 % protein and 11% fat) was introduced and in 1960, 100% of 170 male hybrids, 8–14 months old, revealed multiple hepatomas (HANCOCK AND DICKIE, 1969). Females had no hepatomas at this age but eventually acquired them. More recently, in Australia, a low incidence of hepatomas has been recorded in males of the C3H-A^{vy} and C3H-A^{vy}fB substrains which, in the United States, have a virtual 100% incidence of this lesion (SABINE et al., 1973). At present, it is considered that environmental factors, including diet, bedding and ectoparasitic infestation may be responsible for the reduced incidence; it has already been observed that the replacement of Australian produced feed (Charlick's Mouse Cubes) by United States feed (Old Guilford diet) resulted in significantly higher adult body weights. The major difference between the Australian and American diets is the much higher fat content of the latter.

In the foregoing, consideration has been given only to general dietary effects on hepatoma incidence. We will now consider specific dietary components.

(a) Protein

Mice fed diets containing 9% casein had a significantly lower incidence of benign hepatomas than those fed 18 or 45% casein (RUSCH et al., 1945; TANNENBAUM AND SILVERSTONE, 1949). This effect has been observed in male and female mice of two strains, fed ad lib or isocalorically; it is not dependent on differences in calorie intake or body weight (TANNENBAUM AND SILVERSTONE, 1947, 1949). The differences observed were not due to the amount of dietary protein per se since a 9% casein plus 9% gelatin diet resulted in no higher incidence of hepatomas than a 9% casein diet. However, supplementation of a 9% casein diet with small amounts of the sulphur-containing amino acids methionine and cystine augmented the incidence to equal that observed in mice fed an 18% casein diet (TANNENBAUM, 1953).

(b) Fat

SILVERSTONE AND TANNENBAUM (1951) studied the effect of enriching the fat (partially hydrogenated cottonseed oil) content of the diet from approximately 2–20% on the formation of spontaneous hepatomas in C3H mice and found a small increase of hepatic tumours. In a study of experimental obesity and osteoarthritis, SOKOLOFF et al. (1960) fed diets containing 4·5–60·0% fat (predominantly partially hydrogenated cottonseed oil) to male DBA/2JN, C57L/HeN and STR/N mice from weaning to 72 weeks of age. The strains of mice having the greatest susceptibility to osteoarthritis and obesity (STR/N and C57L/HeN), after receiving the high fat diets, also showed a greater tendency to develop hepatomas. The incidence of hepatomas in the DBA/2JN strain was not increased.

Two groups have studied hepatoma formation in mice in relation to the fatty acid composition of the diet. JARDETZKY et al. (1955), fed 7 groups of C3H male mice, for 54 weeks from weaning, diets containing 17·5% lard, hydrogenated vegetable fat (commercial Crisco) and 5 fractions of the vegetable fat prepared by crystallisation from ether at +15°, +5°, −5° and −15°. Fractions of low melting point (12–26°) produced an incidence of hepatomas much greater than those of higher melting point. No attempt was made to determine the exact composition of individual fractions but, on the basis of analyses by other workers, the high melting point fractions were believed to contain a higher proportion of glycerides of long chain, branched chain and saturated fatty acids and a smaller proportion of unsaponifiable matter. Subsequently, while studying the effects of hydrogenated fats on the growth of the C3H male mouse, KHAN (1957) observed that synthetic fats containing 30–35 % and 10–12 % elaidic acid (*i.e.* the *trans* geometric isomer of oleic acid) not only resulted in improved growth, health and longevity but also increased the incidence of spontaneous hepatomas. This finding appears to substantiate the view expressed by GESSLER (1945) that, during hydrogenation of coconut oil, significant quantities of the *trans* isomer, elaidic acid, may be formed and that this *trans* form may be of significance in modifying hepatoma incidence in mice.

The results of our studies on the effect of diet on the incidence of hepatic parenchymal nodules clearly support much of the published work on this subject. The observed differences in nodule incidence, multiplicity of nodules and nodules per mouse associated with the feeding of stock diet and SSP diet focus attention on the role of diet in general; the differences between mice fed SSP diet containing 5·0 and 10·0 % groundnut oil obviously draw attention to the role of dietary lipid. In turn, this role is more clearly defined by the results of our most recent work in which groundnut oil was added to stock diet and removed from SSP diet. While it is apparent that factors other than dietary lipid are also associated with the development of these hepatic lesions, it is our view that the part played by both the level and the nature of dietary fat is of major importance.

Serum cholesterol

The first report of an association between high plasma levels of cholesterol and cholesterol esters and the development of hepatomas in mice was that of YAMAMOTO *et al.* (1963). High body weight and high plasma levels of cholesterol, cholesterol ester and phospholipids appeared to be genetically associated with the development of hepatomas; mice which were heavier at 12 months of age had a greater tendency to have hepatomas when 16 months old. Unfortunately, the present author was unaware of this work until recently, by which time only a relatively small number of mice fed different diets for 80 weeks was available. Even so, the results obtained are quite striking, serum cholesterol levels in mice fed SSP diet containing 5·0 % groundnut oil being more than twice as high as those of animals fed stock diet or SSP diet without groundnut oil. Comparison of our results with those recorded by BRUELL *et al.* (1962) for five strains of mice shows that serum cholesterol levels in Colworth C57BL mice fed stock diet are somewhat lower than those recorded in C57BL/6JLs-a'a animals, while our results for mice fed SSP diet are very similar to those of C3H mice studied in the United States. The C3H strain is, of course, well recognised as a "high hepatoma strain". Although both BRUELL *et al.* (1962) and YAMAMOTO *et al.* (1963) report that serum cholesterol levels in different strains of mice are genetically determined, the present findings indicate that these levels may be influenced by dietary factors, at least in long-term studies.

Body weight gain

There is a positive correlation between nodule incidence, rapid body weight gain and high terminal body weight. The mechanism and significance of this is unknown.

Hepatic weight

Increase in hepatic weight is frequently reported in association with an increased incidence of nodules, but few observers have considered whether the increase in weight is due to the nodules themselves or to changes in the remainder of the parenchyma. Our observations suggest that the latter plays a significant role and that the increased content of neutral fat in our series is a factor in hepatic enlargement.

Chronic disease

We have observed that hepatic nodule formation is less common in animals with low-grade chronic disease. One such example, *viz.* chronic mite infestation and secondary amyloidosis, has been discussed in relation to Trial 1.

Many other examples have also been noted *e.g.* subacute arteritis, primary intestinal amyloidosis, chronic granulomatous pneumonitis. In many of these instances, mice have been carefully observed over periods of several months, during which time body weight gain has ceased or some loss of weight has occurred. At necropsy and on histological examination, very few hepatic nodules have been identified in such animals and histological hepatic lipid levels have been extremely low, irrespective of the diet fed.

SUMMARY

Throughout much of this communication, the lesions under review and discussion have been designated hepatic parenchymal nodules. Use of this terminology has been deliberate since, in the opinion of the author, terminology commonly used to describe such lesions fails to take account of their varied nature and biological potential. It is considered that the lesions described in this paper represent a broad spectrum covering focal non-neoplastic cellular proliferation in excess of the norm (nodular hyperplasia), benign parenchymal neoplasms (liver cell adenoma) and malignant parenchymal neoplasms (hepatocellular carcinoma). Nodules classified as Type 1 in this paper are probably predominantly of nodular hyperplastic type while those of Type 3 are considered to be hepatocellular carcinomata; Type 2 nodules include lesions of both hyperplastic and benign neoplastic nature.

Failure to appreciate the morphological and behavioural variations in hepatic parenchymal nodules is frequently attributable to selective study of only larger lesions, without consideration of smaller foci and the extranodular pathology of ageing mouse liver. There are many unexplained morphological features in the liver of the older mouse and the possibility that factors which influence the development of these features may also be associated with spontaneous nodule formation has, so far, seldom been considered. Thus, few workers take into account the great differences in metabolic rate among mammals and in particular, the high basal metabolic rate of the mouse. Some of the cytological features observed in mouse liver, *e.g.* polyploidy, binucleate and multinucleate cell formations, intranuclear inclusions, may well be a reflection of adaptive changes. If such be the case, further increases in metabolic load, of nutritional or drug-metabolizing nature, may act as a stimulus to cellular hypertrophy and focal parenchymal hyperplasia. The accumulation of lipid, reported in our studies in mice fed SSP diets, may be an example of such a stimulus. Subsequent progression of a proportion of hyperplastic nodules to a frankly neoplastic state must remain highly debatable. At the present time, differentiation of hyperplastic and neoplastic lesions may be impossible but this is no justification for the inclusion of all hepatic parenchymal nodules in one diagnostic category. Consideration must be given to survival rates, nodular size and multiplicity, behaviour, morphological characteristics and incidence in control and treated animals. If possible, comparisons should be made with positive hepatocarcinogen controls of the same strain fed the same diets.

The results reported in this communication indicate that the increased incidence of nodules associated with the inclusion of certain food additives in the diet of Colworth C57BL mice is attributable almost exclusively to an increased number of hyperplastic lesions under 2–4 mm in diameter; lesions of this type show no histological evidence of neoplasia. Evidence from mice dying/killed before the termination of long-term studies indicated that mortality attributable to hepatic neoplasia was not increased in treated mice and that, in control and treated groups, nodule formation occurred late in the course of the feeding studies. In sharp contrast, dietary inclusion of the known carcinogen, butter yellow, resulted in increased mortality and a high incidence of large, multiple nodules many of which exhibited histological features of malignancy.

Many factors appear to influence the development and incidence of hepatic parenchymal nodule formation and the present studies have highlighted the significance of genetic influence (strain of mouse) (see Chapter 6), animal health and diet; the effect of diet is particularly well defined. The feeding of stock pelleted diet for 80 weeks produced a low level of hepatic nodules, equally distributed between the sexes, in mice which grew relatively slowly, seldom became obese and attained a terminal body weight of approximately 35 g. The use of SSP diets resulted in an increase in nodule incidence, the inclusion of 10% groundnut oil in SSP diet producing a particularly high incidence in females, while both sexes grew rapidly, frequently became obese and attained terminal body weights in excess of 45 g on many occasions. Multiple nodule formation, hepatic weight and hepatic lipid content were greater in mice fed SSP diets.

In conclusion it must be stressed again that an understanding of the nature, aetiology and significance of hepatic parenchymal nodule formation in mice is dependent on an extensive knowledge of the natural history of the lesion in many strains, maintained under different environmental conditions and fed a variety of diets. In such investigations, the utilisation of techniques of proven value in human pathology, clinical biochemistry and transplantation studies is to be commended but we would do well to avoid the use of concepts and terminology applicable to diseases of man until such time as their use is justified and proven. Comparative pathologists are well aware that animal models of human disease are rare and the answer to our present problem will almost certainly be found in the mouse and not in man.

"Disease is from of old and nothing about it has changed; it is we who change as we learn to recognise what was formerly imperceptible...". *(Charcot)*

ACKNOWLEDGEMENTS

The author received much help from many of his colleagues during the preparation of this paper but in particular, wishes to acknowledge the advice and criticism of Drs. Doell, Kirkby, Morris and Wilson, the invaluable assistance of Mr. J. McL. Philp in the preparation of the manuscript and the technical and photographic contributions of Messrs. K. Marlow and A. Shaw.

REFERENCES

AGNEW, L. R. C., AND GARDNER, W. U. (1952) The incidence of spontaneous hepatomas in C3H, C3H (low milk factor), and CBA mice and the effect of estrogen and androgen on the occurrence of these tumors in C3H mice. *Cancer Res.*, 12: 757.
ANDERVONT, H. B. (1950) Studies on the occurrence of spontaneous hepatomas in mice of strains C3H and CBA. *J. Natl. Cancer Inst.*, 11: 581.
BRUELL, J. H., DAROCZY, A. F., AND HELLERSTEIN, H. K. (1962) Strain and sex differences in serum cholesterol levels of mice. *Science*, 135: 1071.
BURNS, E. L., AND SCHENKEN, J. R. (1940) Spontaneous primary hepatomas in mice of strain C3H. A study of incidence, sex distribution and morbid anatomy. *Am. J. Cancer*, 39: 25.
BURNS, E. L., AND SCHENKEN, J. R. (1943) Spontaneous primary hepatomas in mice of strain C3H, IV. A study of intracytoplasmic inclusion bodies and mitochondria. *Cancer Res.*, 3: 697.
COWDRY, E. V. (1955) Modifying factors in cancer development. In: *Cancer Cells*, Chapter 15, pp. 390–430. Saunders, Philadelphia.
DERINGER, M. K. (1959) Occurrence of tumors, particularly mammary tumors, in agent-free strain C3HeB mice. *J. Natl. Cancer Inst.*, 22: 995.
GESSLER, — (1945) In Conference Discussion, *American Association for the Advancement of Science Research Conference on Cancer*, pp. 286–287. F. R. MOULTON (Ed.). Science Press Printing, Lancaster, Pa.
GORER, P. A. (1940) The incidence of tumours of the liver and other organs in a pure line of mice (Strong's CBA strain). *J. Path. Bact.*, 50: 17.
HANCOCK, R. L., AND DICKIE, M. M. (1969) Biochemical, pathological and genetic aspects of a spontaneous mouse hepatoma. *J. Natl. Cancer Inst.*, 43: 407.
HAVEN, F. L., AND BLOOR, W. R. (1956) Lipids in cancer. In: *Advances in Cancer Research*, Vol. IV, pp. 237–314. J. P. GREENSTEIN AND A. HADDOW (Eds.). Academic Press, New York.
HENDERSON, J. F., AND LE PAGE, G. A. (1959) The nutrition of tumours. A review. *Cancer Res.*, 19: 887.
HESTON, W. E. (1963) Complete inhibition of occurrence of spontaneous hepatomas in highly susceptible (C3H × YBR)F$_1$ male mice by hypophysectomy. *J. Natl. Cancer Inst.*, 31: 467.

HESTON, W. E., AND DERINGER, M. K. (1952) Test for a maternal influence in the development of mammary gland tumors in agent-free strain C3Hb mice. *J. Natl. Cancer Inst.*, 13: 167.

HESTON, W. E., AND DERINGER, M. K. (1953) Occurrence of tumors in agent-free strain C3Hf male mice implanted with estrogen-cholesterol pellets. *Proc. Soc. exp. Biol. Med.*, 82: 731.

HESTON, W. E., DERINGER, M. K., DUNN, T. B., AND LEVILLAIN, W. D. (1950) Factors in the development of spontaneous mammary gland tumors in agent-free strain C3Hb mice. *J. Natl. Cancer Inst.*, 10: 1139.

HESTON, W. E., AND VLAHAKIS, G. (1966) Factors in the causation of spontaneous hepatomas in mice. *J. Natl. Cancer Inst.*, 37: 839.

HESTON, W. E., VLAHAKIS, G., AND DERINGER, M. K. (1960) High incidence of spontaneous hepatomas and the increase of this incidence with urethan in C3H, C3Hf and C3He male mice. *J. Natl. Cancer Inst.*, 24: 425.

HUSEBY, R. A., BALL, Z. B., AND VISSCHER, M. B. (1945) Further observations on the influence of simple caloric restriction on mammary cancer incidence and related phenomena in C3H mice. *Cancer Res.*, 5: 40.

JARDETZKY, O., VISSCHER, M. B., AND KING, J. T. (1955) Development of spontaneous hepatoma in mice in relation to composition of dietary fat. *Proc. Soc. exp. Biol. Med.*, 90: 648.

KHAN, N. A. (1957) Effects of tri-elaidin and mixed glycerides of elaidic acid on the growth of the C3H mouse. *Pakistan J. biol. agric. Sci.*, 1: 28.

LIPPINCOTT, S. W., EDWARDS, J. E., GRADY, H. G., AND STEWART, H. L. (1942) A review of some spontaneous neoplasms in mice. *J. Natl. Cancer Inst.*, 3: 199.

McCAY, C. M., ELLIS, G. H., BARNES, L., SMITH, C. A. H., AND SPERLING, G. (1939) Chemical and pathological changes in ageing and after retarded growth. *J. Nutr.*, 18: 15.

McCOY, T. A. (1959) Neoplasia and nutrition. *World Rev. Nutr. Dietet.*, 1: 178.

MILLER, E. W., AND PYBUS, F. C. (1945) The inheritance of cancer in mice with special reference to mammary carcinoma. *Cancer Res.*, 5: 84.

MORESCHI, C. (1909) Beziehungen zwischen Ernährung und Tumorwachstum. *Z. Immunitätsforsch. exp. Ther.*, 2: 651.

MURRAY, R. K., KHAIRALLAH, L., RAGLAND, W., AND PITOT, H. C. (1968) The biochemical morphology and morphogenesis of hepatomas. In *International Review of Experimental Pathology*, Vol. 6. pp. 229–283. G. W. RICHTER AND M. A. EPSTEIN (Eds.), Academic Press, New York.

PHILP, J. McL. (1963) Biological evaluation of glyceran ester PGE 19. In *The Physiological and Nutritional Role of Fats in Human Nutrition*. Wiesbaden Symposium of the International Federation of Margarine Associations, The Hague (Netherlands).

ROWLATT, C., FRANKS, L. M., AND SHERIFF, M. U. (1973) Mammary tumour and hepatoma suppression by dietary restriction in C3H A^{vy} mice. *Brit. J. Cancer*, 28: 83.

RUSCH, H. P., BAUMANN, C. A., MILLER, J. A., AND KLINE, B. E. (1945) Experimental liver tumors. In *American Association for the Advancement of Science, Research Conference on Cancer*, pp. 267–290. F. R. MOULTON (Ed.), Science Press Printing, Lancaster, Pa.

SABINE, J. R., HORTON, B. J., AND WICKS, M. B. (1973) Spontaneous tumors in C3H-A^{vy} and C3H-A^{vy}fB mice: high incidence in the United States and low incidence in Australia. *J. Natl. Cancer Inst.*, 50: 1237.

SILVERSTONE, H., AND TANNENBAUM, A. (1951) The influence of dietary fat and riboflavin on the formation of spontaneous hepatomas in the mouse. *Cancer Res.*, 11: 200.

SILVERSTONE, H., SOLOMON, R. D., AND TANNENBAUM, A. (1952) The influence of natural foods *versus* semi-purified rations on the formation of tumors. *Cancer Res.*, 12: 297.

SOKOLOFF, L., MICKELSEN, O., SILVERSTEIN, E., JAY, G. E. JR., AND YAMAMOTO, R. S. (1960) Experimental obesity and osteoarthritis. *Amer. J. Physiol.*, 198: 765.

STRONG, L. C. (1938) The incidence of spontaneous tumors of mice of the CBA strain after a change of diet. *Amer. J. Cancer*, 32: 80.

TANNENBAUM, A. (1940) The initiation and growth of tumors. Introduction. 1. Effects of underfeeding. *Amer. J. Cancer*, 38: 335.

TANNENBAUM, A. (1942) The genesis and growth of tumors, II. Effects of calorie restriction *per se*. *Cancer Res.*, 2: 460.

TANNENBAUM, A. (1945) The dependence of tumor formation on the degree of caloric restriction. *Cancer Res.*, 5: 609.

TANNENBAUM, A. (1947) Effects of varying caloric intake upon tumor incidence and tumor growth. *Ann. New York Acad. Sci.*, 49: 5.

108

TANNENBAUM, A. (1953) Nutrition and cancer. In: *The Physiopathology of Cancer*, Chapter 15, pp. 392–437. F. HOMBURGER AND W. H. FISHMAN (Eds.). Cassell, London.

TANNENBAUM, A., AND SILVERSTONE, H. (1947) Effect of varying the protein (casein) content of the diet on the formation of tumors in the mouse. *Cancer Res.*, 7: 711.

TANNENBAUM, A., AND SILVERSTONE, H. (1949) The genesis and growth of tumors, IV. Effects of varying the proportion of protein (casein) in the diet. *Cancer Res.*, 9: 162.

TANNENBAUM, A., AND SILVERSTONE, H. (1953) Nutrition in relation to cancer. *Adv. Cancer Res.*, 1: 451.

THORPE, E., AND WALKER, A. I. T. (1973) The toxicology of dieldrin (HEOD). II. Comparative long-term oral toxicity studies in mice with dieldrin, DDT, phenobarbitone, B-BHC and y-BHC. *Food Cosmet. Toxicol.*, 11: 433.

WALKER, A. I. T., THORPE, E., AND STEVENSON, D. E. (1973) The toxicology of dieldrin (HEOD), 1. Long-term oral toxicity studies on mice. *Food Cosmet. Toxicol.*, 11: 415.

WHITE, F. R. (1961) The relationship between underfeeding and tumor formation, transplantation and growth in rats and mice. *Cancer Res.*, 21: 281.

YAMAMOTO, R. S., CRITTENDEN, L. B., SOKOLOFF, AND JAY JR., G. E. (1963) Genetic variations in plasma lipid content in mice. *J. Lipid Res.*, 4: 413.

DISCUSSION

P. M. NEWBERNE. Dietary influences have been overlooked for too long. There are small reports scattered through the literature from about the early 1940s and there was a surge of interest in the early 1950s. Since that time they have been pushed aside and largely ignored. It is findings such as are demonstrated in this paper which indicate that these influences just cannot be ignored. It is well-known that feeds that are mixed for rats and mice and other laboratory animals are mixed in ways similar to those for cattle, swine and chickens. The ingredients of the diet change, for example, the source of protein or fat, depending upon the cost of the ingredient used. For example, if the cost of soyabean meal is greater than another type of protein, the other protein is used. You do not know from one day to the next what is in the feed. We know that there are vast differences in the way that animals respond to different types of protein and fat. Further the vitamins and minerals are not standardized. An example of this is that wheat from central Indiana is virtually deficient in selenium but wheat from the west coast of the U.S.A. may be too high in selenium. Tumour incidence may be drastically altered by dietary influences. In this the response of the rat and the mouse is obviously different as it is possible to induce a dietary cirrhosis in the rat with ease while with the mouse this is done only with extreme difficulty.

GELLATLY. The stock diet we have used has been manufactured by our own company. What you describe does happen, and many of the fluctuating incidences of tumours may be associated with the diet. In our situation the diets are maintained, no matter what the price fluctuations of the ingredients may be. The semi-purified diet is made by us in the laboratory, but even in this there may be variation in the source of the casein used. Casein may vary, and as a result of this we did an 80-week study to investigate a new source of casein. Fortunately, it did not alter the tumour incidence. Concerning lipotrophic factors, the information is very confusing, but it is not possible to compare the rat with the mouse.

P. M. NEWBERNE. There appears to be good correlation of growth in the rapid phase with final tumour incidence. On semi-purified diet and 10% fat diet there is a most rapid growth with a high incidence of tumours. Do you think that this incidence of relating diet to growth rate is a matter of caloric intake?

GELLATLY. At present there is no satisfactory answer. Many factors must be considered, such as metabolic rate. There are many background changes such as increasing ploidy indicating a non-specific stress on the mouse. On this we superimpose a high fat diet. This may have a dramatic effect. There is conflicting evidence of hormonal effects but in our experience, breeding females have a lower incidence of liver nodules than virgin mice.

GRICE. Are you familiar with any work on environmental temperature in modifying tumour incidence?

GELLATLY. I know very few papers describing this, although it has been alluded to.

PURCHASE. Do you consider it necessary to demonstrate metastases in your Type 3 nodules or do you consider them to be carcinoma?

GELLATLY. I do not think that it is necessary to see metastases to diagnose hepatocarcinoma. This diagnosis is based on morphology and in my experience in both mice and other species, an interpretation of carcinoma may be given in the absence of metastases.

Chapter 6

Strain Difference in Natural Incidence and Response to Carcinogens

P. GRASSO AND JOAN HARDY

The British Industrial Biological Research Association, Woodmansterne Road, Carshalton, Surrey (Great Britain)

INTRODUCTION

The mouse has been a favourite animal with cancer research workers for many years, not only because of its small size and prolific rate of reproduction but also because of its alleged sensitivity to carcinogenic agents (TOMATIS *et al.*, 1973). It is undoubtedly true that tumours, particularly of liver, lung, lymphoid and mammary gland tissue, can be readily induced in the mouse by a very large number of carcinogenic agents and some authors have attempted to exploit this sensitivity in order to formulate a bioassay system for carcinogenic activity. The most extensive investigations on these lines were carried out by SHIMKIN *et al.* (1966) and INNES *et al.* (1969). The former treated mice with 29 alkylating agents and evaluated carcinogenic activity on the number of pulmonary adenomas induced over and above the control level; the latter attempted the same type of study by taking into account an increase in the incidence of nodular hepatic lesions which they termed hepatomata.

There is considerable dispute regarding the validity of this type of approach since there are grounds for suspecting that the induction of such tumours may not indicate chemical carcinogenicity (GRASSO AND CRAMPTON, 1972). A variety of reasons have been advanced in support of this contention, the most important of which are: the presence of oncogenic viruses and the unpredictable "background" incidence of the tumours in untreated controls (GRASSO AND CRAMPTON, 1972). The induction of hepatic tumours presents particular problems since, apart from the objections that it shares in common with other types of tumours, there is the added complication of a major disagreement among pathologists regarding the nature of certain nodular lesions (BUTLER, 1971).

In this brief communication it was only possible to deal with a selection of the publications available on the mouse liver tumours. It is hoped, however, that the information presented gives some idea of the natural incidence of nodular lesions in various strains of mice and the ease with which they are induced by carcinogens and other agents. Some information with respect to factors that influence both the natural incidence and response to carcinogens of the adult mouse is also presented and an attempt is made to provide suggestions which might help in establishing some agreement with respect to the pathological interpretation of this lesion.

NOMENCLATURE

The terminology used in describing the nature of the nodular hepatic lesions is not always precise. The term "hepatoma" has been frequently used in this respect but there are grave objections to the use of this term. In the classical sense, hepatoma really means a benign neoplastic lesion made up of liver cells, but by misfortune it has been used widely in human pathology as a shortened version of hepatocellular carcinoma (HUTT, 1971). The meaning of the term hepatoma in experimental cancer research is equivocal and one is never certain whether the writer is using it in the classical sense or in the more popular sense. The terms hepatocellular adenoma or carcinoma are much more explicit.

NATURAL INCIDENCE

Observations on the natural incidence of hepatic tumours in mice are hampered not only by the confusion of nomenclature but also by the relative scarcity of reliable information available. This is particularly so in the case of the early papers (that is those published around 1940). In these publications control groups are either absent or contain very few animals. In some instances only one sex is used, the species or strain is not mentioned, and in others the experiments were terminated too early for hepatoma to develop.

Despite these difficulties, it is possible to form some opinion on the natural incidence of hepatic nodular lesions, often termed "hepatoma", and for the purpose of this communication I have tried to go back as far as I dared to collect data. I thought that the year 1940 was a reasonable one to start with, since by that time design of animal experiments for the testing of chemicals for carcinogenic activity seems to have become reasonably stable even though it is not comparable to present day experiments in terms of animal numbers or in the regard paid to precise details of experimental protocol.

Since the data tend to be presented in a number of styles, it was found necessary to effect some degree of standardization in order to make the data to some extent comparable, and for this purpose expression of the tumour incidence as a percentage seemed to be most appropriate. The percentage was calculated wherever possible on the number of mice surviving to tumour age or number of mice autopsied after week 60 or number of mice killed at the termination of the experiment. In a few instances none of these alternatives was possible and the percentage was calculated on the mice at the beginning of the experiment, in the full realisation that in doing so accuracy had to be sacrificed.

One point needs to be stressed at the outset; the data presented are not exhaustive and many publications had to be omitted. Since the object of the present communication is to present data on sensitivity of strains to carcinogenic agents, as well as data on natural incidence of hepatic tumours, selection has been biased in favour of those publications which reported findings on both control and carcinogen-treated animals.

TABLE I

HEPATIC TUMOURS (HEPATOMAS)

Sub-strain	Number ♂	♀	Incidence % ♂	♀	References
			Strain C3H		
	20	10	20	0	SHIMKIN (1940)
	320	—	26	—	EDWARDS AND DALTON (1942)
	19	—	18	—	SILVERSTONE (1948)
	102	—	85	— ⎫	
f	96	—	71	— ⎬ HESTON et al. (1960)	
e	79	—	78	—	
f	108	—	57	— ⎭	
Y/AʸA	63	—	100	— ⎱ HESTON AND VLAHAKIS (1961)	
Y/Aₐ	94	—	88	— ⎰	
eB/Fe	← 134 →		← 7 →		DAVIS AND FITZHUGH (1962)
AHe	10		30 (20mᵃ)		TAKAYAMA AND OOTA (1965)
eB/De			90	59 ⎱ MURPHY (1966)	
f/He			—	17 ⎰	
HeO	323		32		AKAMATSU et al. (1967)
			Strain BALB/c		
	49	51	Nil		TOTH et al. (1964)
	30	—	Nil	—	CLAPP et al. (1971)
	—	131	—	< 1	TERRACINI et al. (1973)
			Charles River		
	137	144	2	1.5	BIBRA (1971)
	4	4	Nil	Nil	DE MATTEIS et al. (1966)
			Strain A		
	← 400 →		← 1.5 →		EDWARDS et al. (1942)
	← ? →		← < 1 →⎱ ESCHENBRENNER AND MILLER (1945)		
	5	5	0	0 ⎰	
	—	20	—	Nil	SHELTON (1955)
AHe	39	36	7	Nil	KLEIN (1959)
			Strain CF		
CF-W	107	119	Nil	Nil	BIBRA (1969)
CF-W	23	30	Nil	Nil	FREI (1970)
CF-1	125	117	15	Nil	TOMATIS et al. (1972)
CF-1	288	297	20 (0.7mᵃ)	13	WALKER et al. (1972)
			Strain C57		
BL	?10	?10	1	1	KIRBY (1945)
BL	143	171	< 1	< 1	AKAMATSU et al. (1967)
IF	19	31	0	3	CLAYSON et al. (1967)
BL/6/C3H	79	87	10	Nil ⎱ INNES et al. (1969)	
BL/6/AKR	90	82	5	1.0 ⎰	
			Other strains		
Y	← 129 →		← 1.6 →⎱ EDWARDS AND DALTON (1942)		
C	—	150	—	Nil ⎰	

TABLE I *(continued)*

HEPATIC TUMOURS (HEPATOMAS)

Sub-strain	Number		Incidence %		References
	♂	♀	♂	♀	
STS	—	18	—	Nil	MILLER *et al.* (1964)
DBA/2eBDE			—	5	
HR/De			12	6	MURPHY (1966)
Wild Mice			9	3	
CBA/Cb/Se	37	47	11	4	SEVERI AND BIANCIFIORI (1968)
CBA	?10	?10	Nil	Nil	KIRBY (1945)
CBA	285	229	41	27	PYBUS AND MILLER (1942)
ICR	28	—	Nil	—	TAKAYAMA (1969)
RF	262	—	3	—	CLAPP *et al.* (1971)
ASH CS1	429	420	5 (0.2m[a])	Nil	BIBRA (1971)
TF1	107	91	13 (2m[a])	5	BIBRA (1972)
CF-LP	240	240	16 (2m[a])	6	COMMITTEE ON SAFETY OF MEDICINES
BDH-SPF	106	112	2	0	(1972)

[a] m, malignant tumours.

It is hoped, however, that sufficient information has been included to give a fair picture to the reader.

The histological structure of the lesions occurring in untreated animals is not given adequate attention in most of the papers reviewed, although some writers state that the tumours they observed resemble histologically the description of spontaneous hepatomas reported by EDWARDS AND DALTON (1942) and BURNS AND SCHENKEN (1940). These descriptions do not differ remarkably from those mentioned by WALKER *et al.* (1973) and BUTLER AND JONES (Chapter 3) in their detailed description of nodular hyperplasia and hepatic adenoma. The early authors, however, do not lay sufficient emphasis on the type of histological architecture that is associated with malignancy as do the contemporary authors.

Spontaneous malignant lesions, or true hepatocellular carcinomas are much less frequently mentioned than those referred to as hepatomas, and descriptions of these frankly malignant tumours in the literature are even fewer. One is left with the general impression that these malignant tumours are very well differentiated and are usually quite large. Metastasis seems to be uncommon but statements regarding metastasis are really difficult to evaluate since a lot depends on the care with which pulmonary tissue is taken and prepared for histology and on the number of lung sections examined. The fact that metastases have been reported despite these difficulties is important, and suggests that metastasising hepatocellular carcinoma is perhaps not as rare as one is frequently led to believe (Table I).

A first look at the data presented in Table I would show some very large differences in the natural incidence of hepatomas, but a closer look reveals that some strains and sub-strains seem to be particularly prone to the development of these lesions, others less prone (Table I). In this context C3H mice are seemingly highly susceptible to the spontaneous development of these hepatomas. This is particularly so in males. Thus SHIMKIN AND GRADY (1940) reported an incidence of 20% in males, and EDWARDS AND DALTON (1942) and later SILVERSTONE (1948) reported an incidence of 26% and 18% respectively in male mice. The figures of EDWARDS AND DALTON are particularly important since they are based on observations made on 320 male mice. Particular attention continued to be given to male mice of this strain. HESTON et al., as late as 1960 and 1961, reported that the incidence in sub-strains of C3H, designated f, e, Y/A^{y}A, Y/Aa, was as high as 71–100%. MURPHY (1966) also reported an incidence of this order in males of the sub-strain eB/De. This author also gave some information on females of this sub-strain and on f/He sub-strain. This information is particularly valuable because of the scant information available on the hepatoma incidence of C3H females. According to MURPHY, this incidence of hepatoma in female C3H mice varies between 17–59%. Although this is much lower than that of males, it is still considerably higher than one would like to see in untreated animals if it is the intention to use them for carcinogenicity screening tests.

The high incidence in this strain, reported by workers from the United States, is in agreement with that reported by AKAMATSU et al. (1967) who found an incidence of 32% among 323 male mice of the C3H HeO strain. TAKAYAMA AND OOTA (1965) also found an incidence as high as this in their C3H AHe mice but about two-thirds of the tumours were malignant. They are among the few authors to make a distinction between benign and malignant tumours in mouse livers.

There are three other strains of mice with an incidence of hepatoma comparable to that reported for C3H mice: CBA, TF1 and CF-LP. Unfortunately the information available is not nearly as extensive as that for C3H. SEVERI AND BIANCIFIORI (1968) reported a hepatoma incidence of 11% in male and 4% in female mice of the CBA/Cb/Se strain, and ANDERVONT (1950) (Table II) an incidence of 20%. From BIBRA records the TF1 mice appear to be equally susceptible since in roughly 100 males and 100 females an incidence of 13% and 5% of hepatic tumours was found. 2% of the

TABLE II

FLUCTUATING INCIDENCE OF HEPATOMA IN MICE (ANDERVONT, 1950)

Series	Strain	Sex	Number	Tumours %	Year
1	C3H	F	362	11	1942
2	C3H	F	179	5	1943/5
3	C3H	M	43	12	1943
4	C3H	M	86	55	1944
7	CBA	M	68	29	1947
7	CBA	M	40	20	to
7	CBA	F	63	5	1948
7	CBA	F	29	3	

tumours in males had the characteristic adenoid and papilliform pattern suggestive of adenocarcinoma. On about double this number of each sex, CF-LP mice showed an incidence of 16% in males and 6% in females. 2% of the tumours in males were diagnosed as adenocarcinoma (Table I).

In all other strains and sub-strains the incidence is in general 5% or below (Table I), but exceptions exist. Thus a 28% incidence of hepatoma was reported for Strain A mice crossed with He (KLEIN, 1959). CF1 mice also have a high incidence (15–20% in males) but the CF-W sub-strain, in observations conducted on numbers comparable to those of CF1, did not show any spontaneous tumour incidence. These remarkable differences between closely related sub-strains suggest that some genetic or other influences may affect the incidence of these tumours in mice.

It is of some interest to note that wild mice (MURPHY, 1966) also seem to have a high spontaneous incidence. These mice were kept in captivity till the end of their life-span and were fed ordinary laboratory mouse diet, presumably *ad lib*. It is most unlikely that under "wild" conditions mouse diet is anywhere near laboratory fare in either quality or quantity, so that it is not certain to what extent this observation could be taken as an indication of the spontaneous incidence of hepatoma in wild mice under natural conditions.

In all these observations, wherever both males and females were included, the incidence was always greater in males, the proportions varying between 2 : 1 to 4 : 1 but, in some C57BL sub-strains the difference in incidence was even greater. This consistent sex difference points to some possible hormonal factors at work.

An important feature of the incidence of hepatic tumours is the tendency it shows to alter with the passage of time. This is not perhaps unexpected if one compares the percentage incidence of different strains, but when this change occurs in the same strain it cannot fail to attract attention. The figures supplied by MARY TUCKER (personal communication in 1974) of the Pharmaceutical Laboratory of ICI are an example of this. These data show that there is a gradual tendency for the percentage incidence of hepatic tumours of the ICI strain to increase over the years (Fig. 1). An indication that this sort of change could occur in other strains of mice is obtained

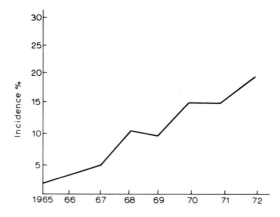

Fig. 1. Hepatic tumours in ICI mice (untreated).

TABLE III

Strain	Weeks				Reference
	Earliest		Mean		
	♂	♀	♂	♀	
C3H	40–50			—	EDWARDS AND DALTON (1942)
CBA/Cb/Se	62	72	86	78	SEVERI AND BIANCIFIORI (1968)
ASH CS1	48	80	78	80	BIBRA (1971)
TF1[a]	73	80	79	80	BIBRA (1972)

[a] Test terminated at 80 weeks.

from the studies of ANDERVONT (1950) which indicate that the incidence of tumours could vary by as much as four times between one year and the next in C3H mice (Table II). This is as yet unexplained but it does show that considerable care is needed in the design of experiments with mice if one hopes to obtain interpretable results.

There is one other point that needs to be mentioned here; the tumour incidence seems to commence between the 50th–60th week. There seems to be agreement from at least 3 sources on this and it is a point worth remembering if one is interested in the early pathology (Table III). No strain differences are apparent here but possibly the studies conducted are too few to show this.

Apart from hepatomas, there are two other types of primary hepatic tumours to which some importance is attached in the literature. One of these is a bile-duct tumour termed cholangioma or cholangio-carcinoma according to the histological appearance. Both these types of tumour occur in mice with the lethal yellow gene (A^y) and with a higher frequency in C3H-A^{vy}fb which have the A^{vy} gene. This latter sub-strain also has a high frequency of benign hepatic nodular lesions and mammary tumours (HESTON AND VLAHAKIS, 1961; VLAHAKIS AND HESTON, 1971). The cholangiomas do not seem to be a particular problem as far as "background" incidence is concerned since their frequency in other strains has not attracted much attention and one must presume that they are only an interesting rarity. COOK et al. (1940) reported that azonaphthalenes and related compounds induced this type of tumour in mice as well as hepatomas. Although some of the hepatomas were successfully transplanted, the cholangiomas uniformly failed to take in mice of the same strain. Other workers confirmed this experience (LEDUC AND WILSON, 1963).

The other type of spontaneous tumour one sees mentioned originates in endothelial tissue. The basic criterion for diagnosing a haemangioma is a proliferative lesion involving endothelial cells which are forming clefts. To be considered a haemangiosarcoma the lesion has to be composed of highly undifferentiated cells forming vascular clefts and invading the surrounding tissue endovascularly, occasionally giving metastases to various organs (TOTH et al., 1964). Haemangiomas and haemangioendotheliomas occur spontaneously much less frequently than tumours of hepatocellular origin.

CHEMICALLY INDUCED HEPATIC NODULAR LESIONS,
INCLUDING TUMOURS, IN THE MOUSE

The long-term administration of a wide range of chemicals to mice by the oral, subcutaneous and other routes, leads to the development of hepatic nodular lesions, some of which are frankly malignant, while others possess a less clear identity as tumours. Since a compound is classified as a carcinogen if it induces a neoplastic response, it is important to distinguish proliferative non-neoplastic lesions from benign and malignant tumours. This distinction is not always possible on histological grounds as many workers in the field admit (SHELTON, 1955; ANDERVONT AND DUNN, 1952; CONFER AND STENGER, 1966; THORPE AND WALKER, 1973) and reading the papers and publications one gets the feeling that the term hepatoma is often used as a screen to conceal this difficulty. Despite the diagnostic difficulties encountered, a number of compounds can be identified as producing an indubitably carcinogenic response in the mouse liver. The morphological descriptions leave little doubt about the malignant nature of the tumour and the number of animals affected in the treated groups is high, yet even at this high level of response certain interesting differences can be observed,

TABLE IV

CHEMICALLY INDUCED HEPATIC TUMOURS IN MICE—DIMETHYLNITROSAMINE

Treatment	Treatment duration (days)	Duration of experiment (days)	Strain	Number	Tumours % Hepato-cell.	Endo.	Reference
50 ppm DW or D	150		ddN	21♂	0	10m	
	150–300		ICR	34♂	6	20m	
	150	To death; average 225–330	C3H	25♂	24b 16m	Nil	TAKAYAMA AND OOTA (1965)
100 ppm DW or D							
	150		ddN	17♂	0	23 m	
200 ppm DW or D	150		ICR	11♂	0	0	
0.001% DW	141	To death 70–630 (max.)	BALB/c	41♂ 46♀	0 0	19b 22m 19b 11m	TOTH et al. (1964)
0.19 mM/kg i.p. once		365	CFW/D	42♀	0	0	FREI (1970)
0.91 mg/kg Daily DW	267- mean	Mean survival time: 360	RF	94♂	2	96m	CLAPP et al. (1971)
1.7 mg/k Daily DW	180	285 (age)	BALB/c	15♂	0	20m	

D, diet.
DW, distilled water.
b, benign.
m, malignant.

not so much in the yield as in the type of tumours induced in various strains by the same compound.

Dimethylnitrosamine (DMN) provides the best example. When administered at high concentrations to BALB/c and ddN mice, they developed haemangioendothelial tumours only. On a similar type of treatment RF and ICR mice developed both haemangioendothelial and hepatocellular tumours (TOTH *et al.*, 1964; TAKAYAMA AND OOTA, 1965; CLAPP *et al.*, 1971) while C3H mice developed only hepatocellular tumours (TAKAYAMA AND OOTA, 1965) (Table IV).

A somewhat similar pattern of response is found after the administration of di-ethylnitrosamine (DEN). Haemangioendothelial tumours only were produced in BALB/c mice (CLAPP *et al.*, 1971) and hepatocellular tumours only were induced in C3H mice (TAKAYAMA AND OOTA, 1965). Both types of tumour were found in FR and ICR strains when given comparable levels of DEN (Table V).

It is not certain, however, to what extent this sort of strain difference is important since it would appear that the type of tumour produced is to some extent dependent on dose levels. Thus, in a dose–response experiment using RF mice, CLAPP AND

TABLE V

CHEMICALLY INDUCED HEPATIC TUMOURS IN MICE—DIETHYLNITROSAMINE

Treatment (daily DW)	Treatment duration (days)	Duration of experiment (days)	Strain	Number	Tumours % Hepatocell.	Endo.	Reference
42 ppm	150	198–204	ICR	11♂	27	9m	TAKAYAMA AND OOTA
	150	198–204	C3H	4♂	100b		(1965)
6 mg/kg	157	270 mean survival	RF	65♂	90	2m	
6.7 mg/kg	151	245, age	BALB/c	73♂	0	23m	CLAPP *et al.* (1971)
3.6 mg/kg	143	285, age	BALB/c	18♂	0	27m	

TABLE VI

CHEMICALLY INDUCED TUMOURS IN RF MICE—DIMETHYLNITROSAMINE
(CLAPP AND TOYA, 1970a)

Treatment (mg/kg)	Duration (days)	Mean[a] survival time (days)	Number	Tumours % Hepatocell.	Endo.
0	0	615	262♂	4	1
1.8	49	450	83♂	0	13
0.4	224	570	17♂	20	0
0.43	406	510	47♂	2	51
0.91	266	360	94♂	0	96

[a] Experiment terminated at death.

TABLE VII

CHEMICALLY INDUCED TUMOURS IN RF MICE—DIETHYLNITROSAMINE
(CLAPP et al., 1970b)

Treatment (mg/kg), cumulative	Treatment duration (days) approx.	Mean[a] survival time (days)	Number (males only)	Tumours %, hepatocell.
0	0	615	162	4
57	9	570	32	17
213	106	387	63	47
321	53	438	30	87
572	50	375	57	98
780	223	291	125	72
943	157	270	64	90

[a] Experiment terminated at death.

TABLE VIII

CHEMICALLY INDUCED HEPATIC TUMOURS IN MICE—
NITROSOPIPERIDINE (I) AND NITROSODIBUTYLAMINE (II)

Treatment (in diet)	Treatment duration (days)	Duration of experiment (days)	Strain	Number	Tumours % Hepatocell.	Endo.		Reference
I 50 ppm	360	360–450	ICR	24♂	25b 8m	12m		TAKAYAMA (1969a)
II 50 ppm	360	360–450	ICR	33♂	30b 15m	Nil		TAKAYAMA (1969b)

TOYA (1970a) induced haemangioendothelial tumours only when they administered DMN at 0.91 mg/kg, and hepatocellular tumours only when they gave approximately half this dose (0.4 mg/kg) (Table VI).

In this experiment CLAPP AND TOYA (1970a) observed that apart from a change in the type of tumour induced, there was also a diminution in the number of tumours (Table VI). This reduction in tumour incidence is roughly proportional to the reduction in dose, providing some indication of a dose–response relationship. A much closer correlation between dose administered and tumour incidence is provided in a dose–response study carried out with DEN (Table VII). The dose–response relationship in this study is in many ways similar to that obtained in rat with DMN and DEN by various workers, notably TERRACINI et al. (1967) and DRUCKREY (1967).

Information about the carcinogenic response of other nitrosamines in mice is relatively scanty, but the few experiments published indicate that tumours of different histogenetic origin might be induced by nitrosamines other than DMN or DEN. Thus, nitrosodibutylamine induces hepatocellular tumours while nitrosopiperidine induces both haemangioendothelial and hepatocellular tumours in ICR mice (TAKA-

TABLE IX

CHEMICALLY INDUCED HEPATIC TUMOURS IN MICE—
URETHANE

Treatment (in diet)	Treatment duration (days)	Duration of experiment (days)	Strain	Nnmber	Tumours % Hepatocell.	Tumours % Endo.	Reference
20 mg × 8 inj.	56	420	C3H	83♂(102)[a]	79b(85)[a]	10(0)[a]	HESTON et al. (1960)
			C3Hf	80♂(96)[a]	90b(27)[a]	10(0)[a]	
			C3He	70♂(79)[a]	91b(78)[a]	7(0)[a]	
0.4% for 20 days	20	c.420	CTM	36♂(88)[a]	2.8b(4.5)[a]	0(3)[a]	DELLA PORTA et al. (1963)
				63♀(99)[a]	6.3b(nil)[a]	4(1)[a]	

[a] Controls

YAMA, 1969a,b) (Table VIII). One presumes that other strains of mice would respond to these and perhaps other nitrosamines by the production of liver tumours of both these histogenetic types.

Urethane provides yet another example of a different response produced by the same chemical carcinogen in different strains of mice. Mice are known to respond to the administration of urethane by developing haemangioendothelial tumours (KIRSCHBAUM et al., 1949; ROE, 1954) and a relatively high incidence of such tumours was induced when urethane was given parenterally in high doses to male C3H mice (HESTON et al., 1960) (Table IX). On the other hand, less tumours were produced in CTM mice than in C3H mice (DELLA PORTA et al., 1963), even though the amount of urethane administered was greater, indicating that CTM mice are less susceptible to tumour induction by urethane than C3H mice.

It is noteworthy that urethane did not increase the incidence of hepatocellular tumours in the experiments with C3H and CTM mice just quoted, but in another experiment INNES et al. (1969) (Table X) reported the induction of this type of tumour only in two sub-strains of C57BL. Thus it would seem that earlier claims that urethane produces specifically tumours of blood vessels only in the mouse liver are only true for certain strains of mice.

o-Aminoazotoluene (o-AT) offers an opportunity of comparing the tumour response in mice of low and high spontaneous incidence. In Strain A mice, this hepatocarcinogen induced an incidence of 82% tumours (SHELTON, 1955). This very high incidence is particularly significant not only because Strain A mice have a low spontaneous incidence, but also because female mice were employed and it is generally accepted that this sex responds less readily than males to the induction of hepatomas by chemical carcinogens. The results of this experiment are in strong contrast to those induced in C3H mice by a single large dose of o-AT. 20 mg injected intraperitoneally once only in males resulted in a 50% incidence of hepatomas. Untreated control mice in this experiment developed a 31% incidence of these tumours so that from this experiment alone one cannot be certain that o-AT is a hepatocarcinogen. It could

TABLE X

CHEMICALLY INDUCED HEPATIC NODULES (HEPATOMAS) IN MICE[a]
(INNES *et al.* (1969) *J. Natl. Cancer Inst.*, 42: 1101)

Chemical	Dose (mg/kg)	Number ♂	Number ♀	Incidence ♂	Incidence ♀	Strain
Urethane	158	20	23	40	52	X
		22	19	64	26	Y
Ethyleneimine	4.64	17	15	88	73	X
		16	11	56	18	Y
Amitrol	1000	18	18	89	100	X
		18	18	89	94	Y
Aramite	464	16	17	38	6	X
		17	16	6	0	Y
Dihydrosafrole	464	17	17	59	0	X
		17	18	47	6	Y
Isosafrole	215	18	16	28	6	X
		17	16	12	0	Y
Safrole	464	17	16	65	100	X
		17	17	18	94	Y
PCNB	464	18	18	11	22	X
		17	17	59	6	Y
p,p'-DDT	46.4	18	18	61	22	A
		18	18	39	6	Y
Mirex	10	18	16	33	50	X
		15	16	33	63	Y
Avadex	215	16	16	81	19	X
		18	15	56	7	Y
bis(2-Chloroethyl) ether	100	16	18	88	22	X
		17	18	53	0	Y
Ethylselenac	10	18	17	67	18	X
		17	17	18	0	Y
ETU	215	16	18	88	100	X
		18	16	100	56	Y
N-(2-Hydroxyethyl)-hydrazine	2.15	17	18	47	6	X
		18	17	56	0	Y
Chlorobenzilate	215	17	18	53	0	X
		17	18	41	0	Y
bis(2-Hydroxyethyl)diethiocarbamic acid K-salt	464	16	18	81	67	X
		17	17	77	18	Y
Strobane	4.46	15	18	13	0	X
		18	18	61	0	Y

X, C57BL/6/C3H/ANF.
Y, C57BL/6/AKR.
[a] Duration 71–83 wk.

be argued that this equivocal response is solely due to the type of treatment and has little to do with the strain of mice employed. This is, however, not quite the case since an identical regimen, using C57BL, a strain of low spontaneous incidence, resulted in the induction of tumours in 25% of treated mice of both sexes compared

TABLE XI

CHEMICALLY INDUCED HEPATIC TUMOURS IN MICE—
OTHER CHEMICALS

Treatment	Treatment duration (days)	Duration of experiment (days)	Strain	Number	Tumours % Hepatocell.	Tumours % Endo.	Reference
o-AT 0.05% D	115	120	A	22♀	82		SHELTON (1955)
2-AAF 0.05% D	up to 420	420	STS	23♀	100b	43m	} MILLER (1964)
OH-AAF	up to 420	420	STS	25♀	100b	36m	
o-AT 20 mg i.p. once only		up to 644	C₃H/HeOs	56♂	50 (31)[a]		} AKAMATSU et al. (1967)
o-AT 20 mg i.p. once only		up to 644	C57/BL	24♂	25 (<1)[a]		
				30♀	26 (<1)[a]		
2-Aminodiphenylene oxide 0.03% D	364 to 469	364 to 469	C57/IF	20♂	10b	60m	} CLAYSON et al. (1967)
				30♀	0b	100m	
4-Aminodiphenyl 0.5 mg 3 × weekly	350	490 approx.	C57/IF	21♂	14b	19m	
				28♀	25b	46m	
Griseofulvine 1% in D	365	365	Charles River	10♂	100		} DE MATTEIS et al. (1966)
				11♀	20		
Izoniazid 2 mg p.d.	252	553 to 623	CBA	18♂	17		} SEVERI AND BIANCIFIORI (1968)
				17♀	12		
Hydrazine sulphate 1.13 mg p.d.	252	483 to 623	CBA	21♂	62		
				21♀	71		

[a] Controls.

with less than 1% in the untreated controls of each sex. This unequivocal carcinogenic response is in keeping with the results from experiments with Strain A mice (Table XI).

The experience with o-AT indicates strongly that mice with a high spontaneous incidence offer no advantage over mice with a low spontaneous incidence in the identification of hepatocarcinogens. In fact, the former could, in a certain sense, lead to considerable interpretative difficulties.

In contrast to the compounds that have been mentioned, DDT produces a fairly uniform tumorigenic response, both in yield and type of tumours in at least 4 strains of mice. INNES et al. (1969) (Table X) reported the induction of a high incidence of hepatomas in males of both C57BL/6/C3H/ANF and C57BL/G/AKR mice which was significantly greater than in the appropriate controls. A similar type of response was observed in females of the former strain, but in female mice of the latter strain

TABLE XII(a)

CHEMICALLY INDUCED TUMOURS IN MICE
(THORPE AND WALKER, 1973)

Treatment (ppm)	Number (CF1) ♂	Number (CF1) ♀	Tumours ♂	Hepatocell.% ♀
Control	45	44	20(4)	23(—)
Dieldrin (10)	30	30	47(53)	40(47)
DDT (100)	30	30	47(30)	47(40)
Phenobarb.(500)	30	28	53(27)	43(32)
β-BHC (200)	30	30	40(33)	30(13)
γ-BHC (400)	29	29	38(55)	34(34)

Duration: 110 wk. ( ), malignant.

TABLE XII(b)

CHEMICALLY INDUCED TUMOURS IN MICE
(WALKER et al., 1973)

Treatment (ppm)	Number (CF1) ♂	Number (CF1) ♀	Tumours ♂	Hepatocell.% ♀
Dieldrin[a] 0	288	297	16(4)	13(—)
0.1	124	90	22(4)	23(4)
1.0	111	87	23(8)	31(6)
10.0	176	148	37(57)	37(55)
ADAB[b] 600	23	21	13(4)	43(38)

Duration: [a] 132 wk; [b] 26 wk. ( ), malignant.

TABLE XIII

CHEMICALLY INDUCED HEPATIC TUMOURS IN CF1 MICE
(TOMATIS et al., 1972)

Treatment (ppm)	Sex	Number	% With tumours Week 0–69	% With tumours Week 70–99
Control	♂	125	Nil	15.0
	♀	117		0.0
2 DDT	♂	126	9.1	39.2
	♀	110	0.0	2.4
10 DDT	♂	111	0.0	56.8
	♀	126	0.0	1.9
50 DDT	♂	135	4.0	46.1
	♀	109	4.2	4.3
250 DDT	♂	117	26.7	96.8
	♀	105	13.8	70.9

TABLE XIV

CHEMICALLY INDUCED TUMOURS IN MICE
(TERRACINI et al., 1973)

Treatment (ppm)	Number ($\female$ BALB/c))	Tumours %	
		Hepatocell.	Endo.
DDT 0	131	0	< 1
2	135	0	< 1
20	128	< 1	< 1
250	121	58	0
DMN 0.0003%	128	< 1	84

the increased incidence of hepatomas was barely significant. The dose administered in this experiment was quite high (equivalent to 200 ppm in diet approximately). THORPE AND WALKER (1973) induced a high incidence of hepatomas by the administration of approximately half this dose of DDT (Table XII) to CF1 mice—the difference in incidence between test and control was not, however, as great as that in the previous experiment. A very similar type of response was obtained in CF1 and BALB/c mice by TOMATIS et al. (1972) (Table XIII) and by TERRACINI et al. (1973) (Table XIV) when amounts of 100 and 250 ppm were added to the diet in life-time studies.

There are some additional features of interest in the tests carried out by TERRACINI AND TOMATIS (see Tables XIII and XIV). Both of these are dose–response studies in which considerable attention was given to the choice of dose levels and to the care of the animals. In both these studies a clear carcinogenic response was obtained only at the highest dose; at the lower dose levels the tumour incidence was no higher than in controls. This is in sharp contrast to the clear dose–response relationship obtained by the administration of DEN in mice (Table VII) and suggests the possibility of a different mechanism of action.

The same sharp rise in tumour incidence was found also by THORPE AND WALKER (1973) in their dose–response study on another widely used chlorinated hydrocarbon insecticide—dieldrin—using CF1 mice. This sudden, rather than gradual, increase in tumour incidence is reminiscent of the type of response observed in another strain of mice—Strain A—when given increasing doses of the simpler chlorinated hydrocarbons CCl_4 and $CHCl_3$ (EDWARDS AND DALTON, 1942; ESCHENBRENNER AND MILLER, 1944, 1945, 1946). Thus it is unlikely that this type of tumorigenic response is peculiar to a particular strain of mice or to a particular chemical. There is some reason for believing that cell injury may be a factor that could account for this sudden increase in tumour incidence.

In both the experiments of TOMATIS et al. (1972) and of THORPE AND WALKER (1973) a proportion of the tumours induced was malignant (Tables XII, XIII), and yet there was no increased mortality or reduced growth rate in mice with malignant liver tumours. This phenomenon is not readily understandable but perhaps loss of weight in mice suffering from malignant tumours is a terminal phase as it is in other species. Since mice experiments are usually terminated after an 80-week treatment the affected mice may be killed before they reach this terminal phase of the disease.

The diversity of experimental conditions used in the testing of other chemicals for carcinogenicity in mice makes it difficult to compare the responses of the strains employed, but there is one extensive piece of work which is an exception. In 1969 INNES *et al.* investigated the carcinogenicity of over 120 chemicals using mouse-hepatoma induction as one bioassay system for carcinogenicity. They employed two strains of mice both, in fact, sub-strains of C57/BL (Table X) and included no less than 7 carcinogens as positive controls. Even at the high doses employed, there was a difference in the response between the two strains of mice which was more marked with some carcinogens than with others. Thus aramite, a hepatocarcinogen in rats, was marginally active only in males of the C57/BL/6/C3H/ANF sub-strain. There was no increased incidence in females of this sub-strain, nor in males or females of C57/BL/6/AKR.

In the case of safrole, males of the former strain responded with a much higher incidence of tumours than males from the latter strain. Females of both strains had an incidence which was very high indeed. In the case of other carcinogens, differences between strains were less marked but were, statistically, significantly higher than controls; however, the marked difference in response with aramite and safrole between the two strains, kept under identical conditions of laboratory housing and diet, raises some doubts about the significance of this type of tumour as an indication of carcinogenic activity. Obviously, factors other than the compound administered seem to be at work and these appear to affect the number of tumours induced.

Hepatoma induction—difficulties in interpretation

The reports summarized in preceding sections do not always give a clear indication of carcinogenic activity. The relatively rare mention of metastases and of the histological features of the hepatic tumours associated with them leads one to conclude, perhaps erroneously, that carcinogenic activity was, in some instances, judged on the induction of nodules which are most probably benign and may even be no more than nodular hyperplasia. The occasional report of liver cell necrosis at stages preceding hepatoma formation suggests that reactive hyperplasia of the nodular type must be constantly kept in mind in evaluating the results. since most of the compounds studied are highly reactive compounds biologically and one would suspect that they might possess a certain degree of hepatotoxicity.

Looking at the results of hepatic tumour induction in the mouse (Tables IX–XIV) with this in mind one would have some difficulty in ascribing carcinogenic activity to a number of compounds if supporting evidence was not forthcoming from other species. Would o-AT or 4-amino-2,3-dimethylazobenzene (ADAB) or hydrazine be classed as carcinogens?

Undoubtedly an empirical correlation between induction of hepatic nodular lesions in the mouse and induction of cancer in other species is important and must be taken into account. From a scientific viewpoint, however, the fact that chemicals, carcinogenic in other species, produce hepatic nodular lesions in the mouse, does not warrant the labelling of a compound of unknown activity as a carcinogen because it produces such hepatic nodules in the mouse. In the absence of data from other species one can only label a compound as carcinogenic in a mouse test if it induces indubitably neoplastic lesions in liver or in other tissues.

Some factors apparently involved in nodule and tumour formation

The tendency for some mice strains, notably C3H and CBA, to develop a high natural incidence of hepatomas, as opposed to other strains in which this lesion appears with much less frequency led to a number of studies on the factors that could account for this difference (ANDERVONT, 1950).

It was soon realized that the incidence in both C3H and CBA mice was not constant but fluctuated from around 0–4% up to 55% (Table II). This changing incidence from year to year was also demonstrated recently in ICI mice (MARY TUCKER, personal communication, 1974) (Fig. 1). At first viruses were thought to account for this fluctuation and investigations were conducted to find out whether the mammary tumour agent could in any way be responsible. A series of observations by ANDERVONT (1950) revealed that this tumour agent is specific for mammary gland tissue and does not influence the formation of these nodules. Despite these observations, one cannot ignore a possible role of some virus in the aetiology of these tumours. Since the studies by ANDERVONT a number of tumour viruses have been identified in mice and one wonders what role these might play in the induction of hepatic nodular lesions including carcinomas. One also wonders whether the mouse hepatitis virus might not be involved in this pathological process.

Hormonal influences also attracted attention as possible aetiological agents and the problem was approached from two avenues. First the influence of breeding and pregnancy was investigated. BURNS AND SCHENKEN (1943) reported an incidence of 27% in 60 breeding C3H males, in contrast to an incidence of 6% in 16 virgins, and an incidence of 0% in 47 breeding females in contrast to an incidence of 10% in 10 virgins. They commented that breeding "favourably influenced the development of tumours in the males and unfavourably influenced the development of tumours in the females". On the other hand, ANDERVONT (1950) found that the percentage incidence in female breeders of the C3H strain varied from 5 to 11% in 170 and 320 animals respectively, an incidence which was comparable to that of virgin mice. Likewise breeding did not affect the incidence in C3H males. A total of 131 breeders showed an incidence of 31·3% and 295 virgins an incidence of 34·9%. Thus the findings of BURNS AND SCHENKEN (1943) could not be substantiated. It is probable that the observations recorded by these authors are unreliable because of the small number of mice on which they were based. Other observers investigated the influence of breeding on hepatoma development (Table XV) and one can conclude that breeding does not appear to influence the incidence of these lesions in either sex of mice.

The second avenue explored involved the possible role of sex hormones since it

TABLE XV

HEPATIC TUMOURS % (HEPATOMAS)—
EFFECT OF PREGNANCY IN CONTROL MICE
(MURPHY, 1966)

Strain	Virgin	Breeder	Force bred
C3HeB/De	59	30	38
C3Hf/He	17	25	
C57BL/He	—	< 1	
DBA/2eBDe	5	—	
HR/De	6	2	
Wild mice	3	4	

TABLE XVI

INFLUENCE OF DIET ON HEPATIC TUMOURS[a] IN MICE
(KIRBY, 1945)

Type of diet	Strain	Number		Number of tumours	
		♂	♀	♂	♀
Full	CBA	6	6	5	4
	C57BL	7	8	5 (1m)	4
Restricted	CBA	4	16	0	0
	C57BL	8	10	1	0

[a] Induced by 4-amino-2,3′-azotoluene.

was universally acknowledged that male mice were much more susceptible to the development of this nodular lesion than female mice. MILLER AND PYBUS (1942) gave weekly subcutaneous injections of 0·05 ml of a 0·06% solution of estrone in olive oil to castrate and intact CBA mice of both sexes and found that under this regimen there was an increased incidence of hepatomas in intact males but a decreased incidence in castrate males as well as in both intact and castrate females compared to the incidence in untreated controls of both sexes. Unfortunately the death rate among the treated animals, including those castrated, was greater than in controls and it is not certain how valid is this interesting observation.

The results of ANDERVONT (1950), however, are slightly more conclusive. Castrate C3H males had consistently lower incidences than did their intact litter mates. Of 183 15-month-old castrates, 11·4% had hepatomas while the incidence of this lesion in 426 intact males of comparable age was approximately 3 times as much (33·8%). This clear difference was not observed in CBA males. In this strain, although castration reduced the tumour incidence the difference was not striking. However, the numbers employed were too small and the results may not be trustworthy, so that one could conclude that the male sex hormones may be involved in some way in the induction of hepatomas.

TANNENBAUM AND SILVERSTONE (1949) used C3H males to study the influence of caloric restriction upon the occurrence of hepatomas and this is discussed by GELLATLY (Chapter 5). There is a limited amount of information on the influence of diet on the chemical induction of hepatomas. SILVERSTONE (1948) reported that rice diet reduced the incidence of spontaneous hepatomas in male mice but this diet did not appear to influence the response to tumour development by o-AT. Restriction of diet, however, did alter response. In an experiment reported by KIRBY (1945) mice were fed the carcinogen 4-amino-2 : 3'-azotoluene contained in a diet made up of 10% casein, 75% boiled potato and salt mixture, baker's yeast and arachis and cod liver oil. This was called a restricted diet presumably because it contained less protein than the standard rat cake diet on which mice were normally fed. The number of tumours found was very much less than in controls fed the standard diet and the same amount of carcinogen. This was true not only for CBA mice reputed to have a high natural incidence, but also in C54 black which is a "low-incidence" strain.

Environmental factors may also influence considerably the incidence of liver tumours and must be borne in mind. C3H-A^{vy} and C3H-A^{vy}fB mice had a very high incidence of hepatic tumours when reared in the U.S.A. On transfer to Australia the incidence of tumours fell dramatically to almost 0%. When the bedding used in the U.S.A. (cedar shavings) was imported into Australia and used for these strains of mice the incidence rose also dramatically to near 100% (SABINE et al., 1973). It is hard to avoid the implication that some factor in the bedding might have been responsible. Although this observation obviously opens up a new avenue for experimentation, it also gives a clear warning against a too facile interpretation of tumour induction and changes in tumour incidence. Before we invoke viruses or genes, perhaps a careful search for some environmental factor, although more mundane, may yield more fruitful results.

Genetic influences have not been studied in detail but the apparent proclivity of mice of the C3H strain, and particularly those carrying the A^{vy} gene, to the development of these lesions leads one to suspect that this is an area worthy of investigation.

Thus there is some evidence that a number of factors may be involved in the induction of this type of tumour, and until more is known about their role it would be unsound to base conclusions on carcinogenic activity on the sole induction of mouse liver tumours, even assuming they are all cancers.

REFERENCES

AKAMATSU, Y., TAKEMURA, T., IKEGAMI, R., TAKAHASHI, A. AND MIYAJIMA, H. (1967) Growth behaviour of hepatomas in o-aminoazotoluene-treated mice in comparison with spontaneous hepatomas. Gann, 58: 323.

ANDERVONT, H. B. (1950) Studies on the occurrence of spontaneous hepatomas in mice of strains C3H and CBA. J. Natl. Cancer Inst., 11: 581.

ANDERVONT, H. B., AND DUNN, THELMA B. (1952) Transplantation of spontaneous and induced hepatomas in inbred mice. J. Natl. Cancer Inst., 13: 455.

130

BURNS E. L., AND SCHENKEN, J. R. (1940) Spontaneous primary hepatomas in mice of strain C3H. A study of incidence, sex distribution and morbid anatomy. *Am. J. Cancer*, 39: 25.

BURNS, E. L., AND SCHENKEN, J. R. (1943) Spontaneous primary hepatomas in mice of strain C3H, II. The influence of breeding on their incidence. *Cancer Res.*, 3: 691.

BUTLER, W. (1971) Pathology of liver cancer in experimental animals. In *Liver Cancer*, WHO/IARC Scientific Publications No. 1, pp. 30–41. International Agency for Research on Cancer, Lyon.

Carcinogenicity Tests of Oral Contraceptives (1972) Report by the Committee on Safety of Medicines. HMSO London, p. 16.

CLAPP, N. K., AND TOYA, R. E. (1970a) The effect of cumulative dose and dose rate on dimethyl-nitrosamine oncogenesis in RF mice. *J. Natl. Cancer Inst.*, 45: 495.

CLAPP, N. K., CRAIG, A. W., AND TOYA, R. E. (1970b) Diethylnitrosamine oncogenesis in RF mice as influenced by variations in cumulative dose. *Int. J. Cancer*, 5: 119.

CLAPP, N. K., TYNDALL, R. L., AND OTTEN, J. A. (1971) Differences in tumour types and organ susceptibility in BALB/c and RF mice following dimethylnitrosamine and diethylnitrosamine. *Cancer Res.*, 31: 196.

CLAYSON, D. B., LAWSON, T. A., AND PRINGLE, J. A. S. (1967) The carcinogenic action of 2-amino-diphenylene oxide and 4-aminodiphenyl on the bladder and liver of the C57X1F mouse. *Br. J. Cancer*, 21: 755.

CONFER, D. B., AND STENGER, R. J. (1966) Nodules in the livers of C3H mice after long-term carbon tetrachloride administration: A light and electron-microscope study. *Cancer Res.*, 26: 834.

COOK, J. W., HEWETT, C. L., KENNAWAY, E. L., AND KENNAWAY, N. M. (1940) Effects produced in the livers of mice by azonaphthalenes and related compounds. *Am. J. Cancer*, 40: 62.

DAVIS, K. J., AND FITZHUGH, O. G. (1962) Tumorigenic potential of Aldrin and Dieldrin for mice. *Toxicol. Appl. Pharmacol.*, 4: 187.

DE MATTEIS, F., DONNELLY, A. J., AND RUNGE, W. J. (1966) The effect of prolonged administration of griseofulvin in mice with reference to sex differences. *Cancer Res.*, 26: 721.

DELLA PORTA, G., CAPITANO, J., MONTIPO, W., AND PARMI, LILIANA (1963) A study of the carcino-genic action of urethan in mice. *Tumori*, 49: 413.

DRUCKREY, H. (1967) Quantitative aspects in chemical carcinogenesis. In *Potential Carcinogenic Hazards from Drugs*, UICC Monograph Series, Vol. 7. RENE TRUHAUT (Ed.), Springer, New York, p. 60.

EDWARDS, J. E., AND DALTON, A. J. (1942) Induction of cirrhosis of the liver and of hepatomas in mice with carbon tetrachloride, *J. Natl. Cancer Inst.*, 3: 19.

ESCHENBRENNER, A. B., AND MILLER, ELIZA (1944) Studies on hepatomas, I. Size and spacing of multiple doses in the induction of carbon tetrachloride hepatomas. *J. Natl. Cancer Inst.*, 4: 385.

ESCHENBRENNER, A. B., AND MILLER, ELIZA (1945) Induction of hepatomas in mice by repeated oral administration of chloroform, with observations on sex differences. *J. Natl. Cancer Inst.*, 5: 251.

ESCHENBRENNER, A. B., AND MILLER, ELIZA (1946) Liver necrosis and the induction of carbon tetra-chloride hepatomas in strain A mice. *J. Natl. Cancer Inst.*, 6: 325.

FREI, J. V. (1970) Toxicity, tissue changes and tumour induction in inbred Swiss mice by methyl-nitrosamine and -amide compounds. *Cancer Res.*, 30: 11.

GRASSO, P., AND CRAMPTON, R. F. (1972) The value of the mouse in carcinogenicity testing. *Food Cosmet. Toxicol.*, 10: 418.

HESTON, W. E., AND VLAHAKIS, G. (1961) Influence of the A^y gene on mammary gland tumours, hepatomas and normal growth in mice. *J. Natl. Cancer Inst.*, 26: 969.

HESTON, W. E., VALAHAKIS, G., AND DERINGER, MARGARET K. (1960) High incidence of spontaneous hepatomas and the increase of this incidence with urethan in C3H, C3Hf and C3He male mice. *J. Natl. Cancer Inst.*, 24: 425.

HUTT, M. S. R. (1971) Epidemiology of human primary liver cancer. In *Liver Cancer*, WHO/IARC Scientific Publications No. 1, pp. 21–29. International Agency for Research on Cancer, Lyon.

INNES, J. R. M., ULLAND, B. M., VALERIO, MARION G., PETRUCELLI, L., FISHBEIN, L., HART, E. R., PALLOTTA, A. J., BATES, R. R., FALK, H. L., GART, J. J., KLEIN, M., MITCHELL, I., AND PETERS, J. (1969) Bioassay of pesticides and industrial chemicals for tumorigenicity in mice: A preliminary note. *J. Natl. Cancer Inst.*, 42: 1101.

KIRBY, A. H. M. (1945) Studies in carcinogenesis with azo compounds, I. The action of four azo dyes in mixed and pure strain mice. *Cancer Res.*, 5: 673.

KIRSCHBAUM, A., BELL, E. T., AND GORDON, J. (1949) Spontaneous and induced glomerulonephritis in an inbred strain of mice. *J. lab. clin. Med.*, 34: 209.

KLEIN, M. (1959) Development of hepatomas in inbred albino mice following treatment with 20-methylcholanthrene. *Cancer Res.*, 19: 1109.

LEDUC, ELIZABETH H., AND WILSON, J. W. (1963) Production of transplantable hepatomas by intrasplenic implantation of normal liver in the mouse. *J. Natl. Cancer Inst.*, 30: 85.

MILLER, ELIZABETH C., MILLER, J. A., AND ENOMOTO, M. (1964) The comparative carcinogenicities of 2-acetylaminofluorene and its *N*-hydroxy metabolite in mice, hamsters and guinea pigs. *Cancer Res.*, 24: 2018.

MILLER, E. W., AND PYBUS, F. C. (1942) The effect of oestrone in mice of three inbred strains, with special reference to the mammary glands. *J. Path. Bact.*, 54: 155.

MURPHY, E. D. (1966) Characteristic tumours. In *Biology of the Laboratory Mouse*. E. L. GREEN (Ed.), Chapter 27, pp. 521–562, McGraw-Hill, New York.

PYBUS, F. C., AND MILLER, E. W. (1942) Incidence of hepatoma in mice of the CBA strain. *19th Ann. Rep. Br. Emp. Cancer Campaign, London*, p. 42.

ROE, F. J. C. (1954) Liver changes in urethane-treated mice appearing after a long latent interval. *32nd Ann. Rep. Br. Emp. Cancer Campaign, London*, p. 170.

SABINE, J. R., HORTON, B. J., AND WICKS, M. B. (1973) Spontaneous tumours in C3H-A^{vy} and C3H-A^{vy}fB mice: High incidence in the United States and low incidence in Australia. *J. Natl. Cancer Inst.*, 50: 1237.

SEVERI, L., AND BIANCIFIORI, C. (1968) Hepatic carcinogenesis in CBA/Cb/Se mice and Cb/Se rats by isonicotinic acid hydrazide and hydrazine sulfate. *J. Natl. Cancer Inst.*, 41: 331.

SHELTON, EMMA (1955) Hepatomas in mice, I. Factors affecting the rapid induction of a high incidence of hepatomas by *o*-aminoazotoluene. *J. Natl. Cancer Inst.*, 16: 107.

SHIMKIN, M. B., AND GRADY, H. G. (1940) Carcinogenic potency of stilbestrol and estrone in strain C3H mice. *J. Natl. Cancer Inst.*, 1: 119.

SHIMKIN, M. B., WEISBURGER, J. H., WEISBURGER, E. K., GUBAREFF, N., AND SUNTZEFF, V. (1966). Bioassay of 29 alkylating chemicals by the pulmonary-tumour response in strain A mice. *J. Natl. Cancer Inst.*, 36: 915.

SILVERSTONE, H. (1948) The effect of rice diets on the formation of induced and spontaneous hepatomas in mice. *Cancer Res.*, 8: 309.

TAKAYAMA, S. (1969a) Induction of tumours in ICR mice with *N*-nitrosopiperidine, especially in forestomach. *Naturwissenschaften*, 56: 142.

TAKAYAMA, S. (1969b) Carcinogenic action of *N*-nitrosodibutylamine in mice. *Gann*, 60: 353.

TAKAYAMA, S., AND OOTA, K. (1965) Induction of malignant tumours in various strains of mice by oral administration of *N*-nitrosodimethylamine and *N*-nitrosodiethylamine. *Gann*, 56: 189.

TANNENBAUM, A., AND SILVERSTONE, H. (1949) The genesis and growth of tumours, IV. Effects of varying the proportion of protein (Casein) in the diet. *Cancer Res.*, 9: 162.

TERRACINI, B., TESTA, MARIA C., CABRAL, T. R., AND DAY, N. (1973) The effects of long-term feeding of DDT to BALB/c mice. *Int. J. Cancer*, 11: 747.

THORPE, E., AND WALKER, A. I. T. (1973) The toxicology of dieldrin (HEOD), II. Comparative long-term oral toxicity studies in mice with dieldrin, DDT phenobarbitone, β-BHC and γ-BHC. *Food Cosmet. Toxicol.*, 11: 433.

TOMATIS, L., TURUSOV, V., DAY, N., AND CHARLES, R. T. (1972) The effect of long-term exposure to DDT on CF-1 mice. *Int. J. Cancer*, 10: 489.

TOMATIS, L., PARTENSKY, C., AND MONTESANO, R., (1973) The predictive value of mouse liver tumour induction in carcinogenicity testing—a literature survey. *Int. J. Cancer*, 12: 1.

TOTH, B., MAGEE, P. N., AND SHUBIK, P. (1964) Carcinogenesis study with dimethylnitrosamine administered orally to adult and subcutaneously to newborn BALB/c mice. *Cancer Res.*, 24: 1712.

VLAHAKIS, G., AND HESTON, W. E. (1971) Spontaneous cholangiomas in strain C3H-A^{vy}fB mice and in their hybrids. *J. Natl. Cancer Inst.*, 46: 677.

WALKER, A. I. T., THORPE, E., AND STEVENSON, D. E. (1973) The toxicology of dieldrin (HEOD), I. Long-term oral toxicity studies in mice. *Food Cosmet. Toxicol.*, 11: 415.

DISCUSSION

BUTLER. In assessing strain differences, there is, as you mention, a report [SABINE *et al.* (1973) *J. Natl. Cancer Inst.*, 50: 1237] of an inbred strain of mice in which when transferred to another laboratory the incidence of both liver and mammary tumours was reduced. Is there any good evidence that the strain differences which have been described are genetically determined?

GELLATLY. This is one possible example of the many factors of diet, bedding, and there are other examples of a changing incidence of a neoplasm within the same strain. The effects of these environmental factors is enormous. It is also well-known that when one is interested in a lesion, it becomes more common. We have therefore standardized our post mortem techniques to remove operator bias in this. Another factor is the breeding of animals. Is the selection for breeding the same when the staff are changed? I would consider that there are strain differences in response to chemicals; for example, when the same diet and compound are fed C3H mice respond differently from CBA mice. It is possible that this is a genetic effect but this may be an increase in body weight which modifies the incidence of hepatic neoplasia. Otherwise there does not appear to be good evidence that there is a direct genetic link with incidence of hepatic neoplasia.

REUBER. A consideration arising from Dr. GRASSO's paper is a problem of dose–response relationship. It is important to distinguish between hyperplasia and carcinoma in assessing a dose response. Also it is necessary to take into account both the number and size of the carcinomas.

GRASSO. It is also necessary to emphasize the duration of the experiment. Obviously, this will modify any dose–response relationship.

GELLATLY. Another factor comes into the problem of dose response when dealing with strains of a high incidence. The first spontaneous nodules tend to appear between 50–70 weeks and if an 80-week study is performed by the time the mice reach 50–60 weeks of age, intercurrent disease begins to play an important part in tumour incidence. In our mice, where there has been a cessation of body weight gain as a result of chronic non-neoplastic disease, when finally examined the livers seldom show nodules. These effects occur late in any test and may modify dose–response relationships.

GRASSO. It is also our observation that mice which exhibit generalized toxic reaction to a compound causing reduction in body weight gain tend to have a lower incidence of liver tumours and indeed other neoplasms although survival has not been altered.

J. W. NEWBERNE. I think that the data on DDT body weight changes are interesting. There is a general feeling among toxicologists that one must demonstrate some adverse effect such as reduction in body weight gain or some gross change. This would be difficult to do with DDT. What index would you recommend in order to demonstrate highest tolerated dose which is a system which has been recommended?

GRASSO. We have our doubts whether the maximum tolerated dose (MTD) is a suitable dose. We have studied safrole with this in mind, and have difficulty in assessing a maximum tolerated dose, as a short-term MTD may be different from a long-term figure as a result of enzyme induction. As induced enzymes appear to degrade, the only way to design experiments using the maximum tolerated dose is to repeat the experiment after one's initial experience.

P. M. NEWBERNE. In testing a compound how do you determine the dose levels to be used? Usually we go to a high dose which produces an effect such as weight reduction then reduce it stepwise. However, what is the proper approach?

GRASSO. I do not know what is the proper approach. At BIBRA we do a 90-day test to get some preliminary information to find out at what levels we might get pathological changes. For a long-term carcinogenicity test our top dose level is that which might produce only slight effect and then use lower doses as well.

J. W. NEWBERNE. There are examples of steroid inhibitors which produce marked liver hypertrophy. In two incidences at levels which produce a 10% increase in liver weight, there were no long-term effects over 18–20 months. At doses which produced a 20–30% increase in liver weight, nodules and other non-proliferative changes were seen. Realistically the compounds will never be used in this way. The interpretation of these results is that the hepatic systems involved in enzyme induction may be overwhelmed and then one is dealing with a stressed situation. It is obviously difficult to generalize and lay down any rules but it is necessary to examine each case.

Chapter 7

Neonatal Induction of Hepatic and Other Tumours

FRANCIS J. C. ROE

4, Kings Road, Wimbledon
London SW19 8QN
(Great Britain)

In 1961 we reported the results of our first experience of the consequences of injecting a known carcinogen into newborn mice (ROE et al., 1961). We had been stimulated to undertake this experiment by a report of PIETRA et al. (1959) which described an increased incidence of malignant lymphoma and lung adenomas in mice given 30 μg 7,12-dimethylbenz(a)anthracene (DMBA) at birth by subcutaneous injection. We repeated their experiment using "101" strain and CBA strain mice instead of Swiss albino mice. In mice killed after one year, as expected from their results, we observed an increased incidence of malignant lymphoma and lung tumours. We also saw, mainly in DMBA-treated mice, neoplasms of a variety of other sites including the liver (Table I). We were in fact hesitant to record our data in respect of liver tumours, the number of animals affected was low, even in the CBA strain; furthermore, such tumours are commonly found in untreated mice older than 52 weeks. Also the response in terms of liver tumours was trivial in comparison with that of tumours of the lungs and of the lymphoreticular system. However, two features of the response of the liver were recorded that conform to a general pattern which is now clear. Firstly, although approximately equal numbers of males and females were at

TABLE I

LIVER-CELL TUMOURS AND LUNG TUMOURS IN "101" STRAIN AND CBA STRAIN MICE GIVEN 30 μg DMBA IN AQUEOUS GELATIN BY SUBCUTANEOUS INJECTION AT BIRTH (ROE et al., 1961)

Group	Treatment	Strain	Number of mice examined post-mortem[a]	Number with lung tumours	Average lung tumours per per tumour-bearing mouse	Number with liver tumours[a]	Average liver tumour per tumour-bearing mouse
1	DMBA/gelatine	CBA	18	16	14	3	> 10
2	Gelatine	CBA	25	0	0	1	1
3	None	CBA	39	3	2	2	1.5
4	DMBA/gelatine	"101"	25	24	14	1	4
5	None	"101"	40	6	2	1	1

[a] In each group there were approximately equal numbers of males and females, but all except one of the mice with liver cell tumours (Group 2) were males.

134

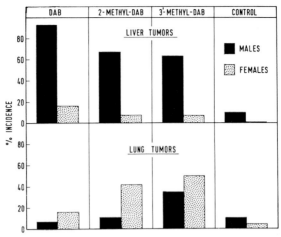

Fig. 1. Incidence of liver and lung tumours in mice killed between 52 and 54 weeks after exposure at birth to 5×200 μg doses of DAB, 2-methyl-DAB, 3'-methyl-DAB or the vehicle, arachis oil, only (treatments given by subcutaneous injection on each of the first five days of life).

TABLE II

LIVER CELL NEOPLASMS IN MICE TREATED WITH DAB AND ITS DERIVATIVES KILLED AT END OF EXPERIMENT

Group	Treatment	Sex	Number killed at end of experiment	Percent with liver tumours	Percent with multiple liver tumours	Average number of liver tumours per survivor
A	DAB	♂	28	92	86	2.0
		♀	25	16	12	0.3
B	2-Methyl-DAB	♂	27	67	44	2.0
		♀	24	8	4	0.1
C	3'-Methyl-DAB	♂	38	63	47	1.6
		♀	14	7	0	0.1
D	Arachis oil only	♂	31	10	7	0.3
		♀	25	0	0	0

risk, all except one of the 8 that developed liver-cell tumours were males. Secondly, the apparently more striking effect of DMBA treatment was to increase the multiplicity of liver tumours in the few animals that bore them rather than to increase the proportion of mice that developed them. This was especially striking in the CBA strain. We have repeatedly encountered both these features in numerous studies in other strains of mice since 1961. A third feature of the findings of our 1961 study was the presence of eosinophilic cytoplasmic inclusions similar to those described by BURNS AND SCHENKEN (1940). These have been observed mainly in C3H strain mice by CRAIGIE (1955). It is my impression, but only an impression, that inclusions of this kind are now found less frequently in both C3H and CBA strain mice. It is certainly true that we are rarely seeing such inclusions in liver cell tumours in Swiss mice today.

More recently, we reported the results of a study in which 4-dimethylaminoazo-benzene (DAB) or its 2-methyl or 3'-methyl derivatives were given to mice at birth (ROE *et al.*, 1971). The results are summarised in Fig. 1 and Table II. Treatment consisted of 5 doses of 200 µg of each test substance in arachis oil on each of the first 5 days of life. Control mice were given arachis oil only. Treatment with all three substances was associated with a significant increase in incidence of liver cell tumours in males, the effect being greatest with DAB itself. A slightly increased incidence in females was not statistically significant. Lung tumours were also seen in significant excess in response to the two methylated derivatives but not to DAB itself. It is

TABLE III

LIVER AND LUNG TUMOURS IN MALE SWISS MICE GIVEN BENZ(A)ANTHRACENE OR ITS K-REGION EPOXIDE AT BIRTH

Compound	Dose given on days 0, 1 and 2 (µg)[a]	Tumour incidence at 70 weeks				
		Number of mice	Mice with liver tumour	Mice with > 1 liver tumour	Mice with lung tumour	Mice with > 1 lung tumour
B(a)A	200	15	15	15	4	4
	100	19	15	11	5	3
	50	25	9	5	5	2
B(a)A epoxide	200	18	5	4	2	1
	100	26	12	8	3	0
	50	16	4	1	5	1
Vehicle (PEG 400) only		22	4	0	3	1

[a] By subcutaneous injection of dose in 0.02 ml PEG 400.

TABLE IV

LIVER AND LUNG TUMOURS IN FEMALE SWISS MICE GIVEN BENZ(a)ANTHRACENE OR ITS K-REGION EPOXIDE AT BIRTH

Compound	Dose given on days 0, 1 and 2 (µg)[a]	Tumour incidence at 70 weeks				
		Number of mice	Mice with liver tumour	Mice with > 1 liver tumour	Mice with lung tumour	Mice with > 1 lung tumour
B(a)A	200	18	2	1	10	10
	100	13	0	0	5	2
	50	21	2	1	7	3
B(a)A epoxide	200	20	2	0	1	0
	100	22	0	0	6	5
	50	16	0	0	2	0
Vehicle (PEG 400) only		23	1	0	1	2

[a] By subcutaneous injection of dose in 0.02 ml PEG 400.

TABLE V

LIVER AND LUNG TUMOURS IN MALE SWISS MICE GIVEN CHRYSENE OR 7-METHYLBENZ(a)ANTHRACENE OR THEIR K-REGION EPOXIDES AT BIRTH

Compound	Dose given on days 0, 1 and 2 (μg)	Tumour incidence at 70 weeks				
		Number of mice	Mice with liver tumour	Mice with > 1 liver tumour	Mice with lung tumour	Mice with > 1 lung tumour
7-MethylB(a)A	100	23[a]	12	12	13	11
7-MethylB(a)A epoxide	100	20	4	2	2	2
Chrysene	100	27	13	6	1	1
Chrysene epoxide	100	21	8	3	0	0
Vehicle (PEG 400) only		30	9	1	3	1

[a] 10 of the mice with lung tumours and 11 of those with liver tumours died between 50 and 70 weeks.

TABLE VI

LIVER AND LUNG TUMOURS IN FEMALE SWISS MICE GIVEN CHRYSENE OR 7-METHYLBENZ(a)ANTHRACENE OR THEIR K-REGION EPOXIDES AT BIRTH

Compound	Dose given on days 0, 1 and 2 (μg)	Tumour incidence at 70 weeks				
		Number of mice	Mice with liver tumour	Mice with > 1 liver tumour	Mice with lung tumour	Mice with > 1 lung tumour
7-MethylB(a)A	100	10	0	0	1	1
7-MethylB(a)A epoxide	100	22	0	0	6	3
Chrysene	100	21	0	0	1	0
Chrysene epoxide	100	20	1	0	0	0
Vehicle (PEG 400) only		15	0	0	1	0

interesting (Table II) to note that liver tumours tended to be multiple in the mice that bore them.

In other studies in collaboration with Dr. P. GROVER, Dr. P. SIMS and Mr. B. C. V. MITCHLEY (1975), we examined the effects of exposing newborn mice to benz-(a)anthracene, chrysene and 7-methyl(a)anthracene and their respective K-region epoxides (see Tables III–VI). Previous *in vitro* studies tended to support the hypothesis (GROVER *et al.*, 1971, 1972; KEYSELL *et al.*, 1973) that the carcinogenicity of polycyclic hydrocarbons is secondary to the formation from them of K-region epoxides (GROVER *et al.*, 1971; MARQUARDT *et al.*, 1972; HUBERMAN *et al.*, 1972). *In vivo* studies in adult animals, however, have all indicated the epoxides to be less active than the parent compounds. The results of our studies in newborn mice are for the main part consistent with those of other *in vivo* studies. Benz(a)anthracene and 7-methylbenz(a)anthracene were both more active in increasing both liver tumours and lung tumours than their respective K-region epoxides. Chrysene and its K-region epoxide both increased the incidence of liver tumours but not of lung tumours. Studies

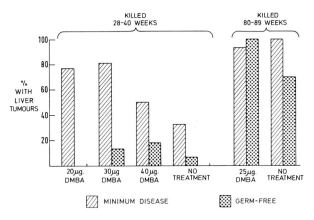

Fig. 2. Effect of various doses of DMBA given at birth on germ-free and minimum disease conventionally maintained male C3H mice killed at 28–40 weeks or 80–89 weeks.

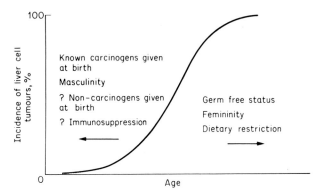

Fig. 3. Factors known to influence the age at which liver-cell tumours develop in C3H mice.

involving other routes of administration and other species had led most earlier investigators to regard chrysene as probably non-carcinogenic (CLAYSON, 1962) and benz(a)anthracene as being on the borderline (STEINER AND FALK, 1951). 6-Aminochrysene is also of interest in this context. We (ROE et al., 1969) found that when this substance was given at birth to male Swiss mice, an increased number of both liver and lung tumours developed. This was not seen in female mice. Tests for carcinogenicity in adult rats and mice have given consistently negative results (RUDALI et al., 1953; LAMBELIN et al., 1967). As we noted in our earliest study of this kind (ROE et al., 1961), liver tumours were multiple in the animals in which they occur and yet did not arise at all in a proportion of similarly treated mice.

In our study in 1970 (ROE AND GRANT, 1970), we reported that liver cell tumours were present in 100% of untreated male C3H mice maintained under conventional conditions and in 70% of comparable mice kept germ-free after 80–90 weeks. By comparison less than 10% of conventional or germ-free females of similar age had such tumours. Exposure of germ-free males to DMBA at birth brought liver tumour incidence up to 100% by age 80–90 weeks. In females, whether germ-free or conventional, similar treatment with DMBA increased liver tumour incidence to about 50% of animals (Figs. 2 and 3). These results also indicate that it is important to consider the age-related incidence. If the 28–40-week group is considered separately one might conclude that germ-free status protected the animals against tumour induction.

Although, on the basis of extensive evidence involving many different species and tissues, I have no doubt that DMBA itself (or a metabolite derived from it) is capable of inducing cancer (*i.e.* is a true carcinogen). I do not believe it is reasonable to conclude from the results of our experiments in C3H mice that DMBA induces liver-cell tumours in that strain. The kinds of liver tumour seen in young DMBA-treated mice were exactly the same as those seen in untreated older animals. The tumours seen relatively infrequently in young DMBA-treated germ-free mice were seemingly exactly the same as those seen relatively more frequently in young DMBA-treated conventionally maintained mice.

The histological characteristics of the liver-cell tumours which arise in response to chemicals given to mice at birth are similar to those of spontaneously occurring tumours and are described in Chapter 3. Some lesions are difficult to distinguish from normal liver parenchyma. Their distinguishing features may be no more than a slight difference in staining affinity (usually more basophilic), a small difference in average cell size, somewhat more (or less) fatty degeneration than surrounding liver parenchyma, and loss of lobular structure. It is, I am sure, incorrect to regard such lesions as "hyperplastic nodules" since there is no evidence, in terms of high mitotic counts or high rates of cell turnover, that they are hyperplastic. These lesions do not appear to be invasive and do not, in my experience metastasise. However, they are found more often in the livers of animals that have undoubted liver neoplasms than in the livers of animals without such neoplasms. I believe, therefore, that they are probably benign neoplasms.

RICE (1973) reported the results of a study on transplacental exposure in which pregnant C3H mice were given 1-ethyl-1-nitrosourea (ENU). The male offspring developed large numbers of liver and lung tumours and the females many lung but few liver tumours. Gonadectomy and treatment with oestrogen dramatically reduced the incidence of liver but not lung tumours in male offspring. Gonadectomy and treatment with androgen was associated with a 5-fold increase in liver tumour incidence in female offspring but was without effect on lung tumour incidence.

RICE (1973) states that malignant liver-cell tumours are rare in his strain of C3H mice and that hepatoblastomas of kinds that he does not see in untreated mice arose in the male offspring of mice exposed to ENU on about the 12th day of gestation. In my experience, malignant liver-cell tumours occur not infrequently spontaneously in mice of various strains and there is nothing unique about the tumours he illustrates as occurring in mice exposed transplacentally to ENU.

All in all, RICE's (1973) findings suggest that the susceptibility of newly born mice to agents which enhance liver-cell tumour development is shared by foetuses still *in utero*, and that factors which influence liver tumour development in response to post-natal stimuli act also in the case of liver tumours arising in response to prenatal stimuli.

In our 1961 paper, we suggested that the injection of test chemicals into newborn mice might be a useful method for screening for carcinogenicity. Since that time, I have grown increasingly uneasy about the value of the method. From the start it was clear that even potent carcinogens could give negative results in such tests. This fact has led Regulatory Bodies to reject negative evidence from newborn mouse studies as a substitute for conventional life-span carcinogenicity tests on more mature animals. The problem that persists is that some workers are inclined to accept positive results from newborn mouse studies as proof, or strong evidence, of carcinogenic potential. In view of all the knowledge that we now have about factors which influence the incidence of malignant lymphoma, lung tumours and liver tumours in mice, it would seem today to be wholly unwise to accept increased incidence of any of these kinds of neoplasm, by itself, as indicative of cancer inducing activity.

The interpretation of liver tumorigenesis in mice

It is clear to me that many substances which are unquestionably capable of inducing cancers in other species or tissues can increase the risk of development of liver-cell tumours in mice and that the effect is much more readily produced in males than in females. It is not established that the extra liver tumours that appear are directly induced by the substances concerned or whether some other mechanism is involved. My doubts regarding the interpretation of liver-cell tumorigenesis in mice do not concern the nature of the lesions; the majority of them are undoubtedly neoplastic and a significant proportion of them, especially in older mice, are unquestionably malignant. The possibility that other non-specific mechanisms may be involved has to be seriously entertained since germ-free status, sex and dietary intake (Table VII) all have been shown to markedly effect the age-standardised incidence of liver-cell tumours in otherwise untreated mice. This is summarised in Fig. 3. It is my opinion,

TABLE VII

EFFECT OF DIETARY INTAKE ON INCIDENCE OF LIVER, LUNG AND OTHER TUMOURS IN SWISS MICE[a]
(Data from Miss M. TUCKER, ICI Laboratories, Alderley Park)

Group	Number of mice	Feeding[b]	Total tumours by 18 months	Liver tumours	Lung tumours	Lymphoreticular neoplasms	Other neoplasms
1	40	4 g diet/day 1 mouse/cage	4	1	1	2	0
2	40	5 g diet/day 1 mouse/cage	4	2	0	1	1 testis
3	40	Diet ad lib. 1 mouse/cage	32	15	2	11	2 testes 1 kidney 1 thyroid
4	40	Diet ad lib. 5 mice/cage	23	8	6	9	0

[a] Outbred Swiss albino males maintained under SPF conditions.
[b] Standard pelleted diet.

therefore, that the demonstration that a substance can, on administration to neonatal mice, increase the incidence of liver-cell tumours is insufficient evidence to label the compound a carcinogen for the mouse or any other species. I regard it as important and perhaps urgent that we should know more about why mice develop liver-cell tumours apparently spontaneously. In particular why do mice of some strains develop such lesions in very high incidence? What is the explanation of the sex difference? How can slight differences in dietary intake have disproportionately large effects on tumour incidence? These fundamental questions deserve priority in our research. Only when we have clear answers to them will we be able with confidence to interpret experiments in which tumours of the same kinds arise excessively in apparent response to exposure to test substances.

SUMMARY

The exposure of mice to certain chemicals during the neonatal period is associated with increased incidence of liver-cell neoplasms. Males are more susceptible than females. The tumours are histologically similar to those seen in untreated animals. In some strains where there is a 100% incidence in old age, it is difficult to know whether the tumours which arise early are indeed induced or rather represent enhancement of another factor. These findings suggest that an increased incidence of liver-cell tumours in mice exposed at birth to a chemical compound is not a reliable indication that the compound is a carcinogen. So far, there is no evidence that prenatal exposure to a compound may give a fundamentally different outcome as far as liver tumour incidence is concerned than postnatal exposure to the same agent.

REFERENCES

BURNS, E. L., AND SCHENKEN, J. R. (1940) Spontaneous primary hepatomas in mice of strain C3H: A study of incidence, sex distribution and morbid anatomy. *Am. J. Cancer*, 39: 25.

CLAYSON, D. B. (1962) *Chemical Carcinogenesis*, pp. 142-143. Churchill, London.

CRAIGIE, J. (1955) Spontaneous hepatomas in mice. *Ann. Rept. Imp. Cancer Res. Fund*, 52: 8.

GROVER, P. L., SIMS, P., HUBERMAN, E., MARQUARDT, H., KUROKI, T., AND HEIDELBERGER, C. (1971) *In vitro* transformation of rodent cells by K-region derivatives of polycyclic hydrocarbons. *Proc. Natl. Acad. Sci. (U.S.)*, 68: 1098.

GROVER, P. L., HEWER, A., AND SIMS, P. (1972) Formation of K-region epoxides as microsomal metabolites of pyrene and benzo(a)pyrene. *Biochem. Pharm.*, 21: 2713.

GROVER, P. L., SIMS, P., MITCHLEY, B. V. C., AND ROE, F. J. C. (1975) The carcinogenicity of polycyclic hydrocarbon epoxides in newborn mice. *Brit. J. Cancer*, 31: 182.

HUBERMAN, E., KUROKI, T., MARQUARDT, H., SELKIRK, J. K., HEIDELBERGER, C., GROVER, P. L., AND SIMS, P. (1972) Transformation of hamster embryo. *Cancer Res.*, 32: 1391.

KEYSELL, G. R., BOOTH, J., GROVER, P. L., HEWER, A., AND SIMS, P. (1973) The formation of "K-region" epoxides as hepatic microsomal metabolites of 7-methylbenz(a)anthracene and 7,12-dimethylbenz(a)anthracene and their 7-hydroxymethyl derivatives. *Biochem. Pharm.*, 22: 2853.

LAMBELIN, G., MEES, G., AND BUU-HOI, N.P. (1967) Chronic toxicity studies on 6-aminochrysene in the rat. *Arzneimittel-Forsch.*, 17: 1117.

MARQUARDT, H., KUROKI, T., HUBERMAN, E., SELKIRK, J. K., HEIDELBERGER, C., GROVER, P. L., AND SIMS, P. (1972) Malignant transformation of cells derived from mouse prostate by epoxides and other derivatives of polycyclic-hydrocarbons. *Cancer Res.*, 32: 716.

PIETRA, G., SPENCER, K., AND SUBIK, P. (1959) Response of newly born mice to a chemical carcinogen. *Nature*, 183: 1689.

RICE, J. M. (1973) The biological behaviour of transplacentally induced tumours in mice. In: *Transplacental Carcinogenesis*, L. TOMATIS, U. MOHR AND W. DAVIS (Eds.), I.A.R.C. Scientific Publication No. 4, pp. 71–83.

ROE, F. J. C., AND GRANT, G. A. (1970) Inhibition by germ-free status of development of liver and lung tumours in the mice exposed neonatally to 7,12-dimethylbenz(a)anthracene: implications in relation to tests for carcinogenicity. *Int. J. Cancer*, 6: 133.

ROE, F. J. C., ROWSON, K. E. K., AND SALAMAN, M. H. (1961) Tumours of many sites induced by injection of chemical carcinogens into newborn mice. A sensitive test for carcinogenesis: The implications for certain immunological theories. *Brit. J. Cancer*, 15: 515.

ROE, F. J. C., CARTER, R. L., AND ADAMTHWAITE, S. (1969) Induction of liver and lung tumours in mice by 6-aminochrysene administered during the first three days of life. *Nature*, 221: 1063.

ROE, F. J. C., WARWICK, G. P., CARTER, R. L., PETO, R., ROSS, W. C. J., MITCHLEY, B. C. V., AND BARRON, N. A. (1971) Liver and lung tumours in mice exposed at birth to 4-dimethylaminoazobenzene or its 2-methyl or 3′-methyl derivatives. *J. Natl. Cancer Inst.*, 47: 593.

RUDALI, G., BUU-HOI, N. P., AND LACASSAGNE, A. (1953) Sur quelques effets biologiques du 2-aminochrysène. *Compt. Rend.*, 236: 2020.

STEINER, P. E., AND FALK, H. L. (1951) Summation and inhibition effects of weak and strong carcinogenic hydrocarbons: 1,2-benzanthracene, chrysene, 1,2,5,6-dibenzanthracene, and 20-methylcholanthrene. *Cancer Res.*, 11: 56.

DISCUSSION

GRICE. From the standpoint of testing agencies, both the foetus and the neonate are exposed to many compounds. Greater concern for this has come about from the suggestion, arising from the saccharin studies that saccharin or one of its metabolites may be carcinogenic, when the foetus is exposed to it. The two positive studies of the eight which have been reported with saccharin, used both *in utero* and post-natal exposure whereas the six negative studies used exposure only in adults. Therefore, the transplacental route should be used in carcinogenicity studies where the foetus may be exposed. However, I would much prefer to use the rat rather than the mouse for this type of experiment.

LEONARD. If the proximate carcinogen is a metabolite of the compound administered, the maturity of the metabolic processes in the foetus and the neonate may result in a negative result.

P. M. NEWBERNE. There is increasing concern over pre- and peri-natal exposure to compounds. I have a feeling that some are trying to produce cancer in any way possible as they are interested in the tumour, which may of course be correct if their interest lies in the field of metabolism. But treating animals in this way to determine whether compounds are of concern to public health is a different matter. We know little of the factors concerned in the liver of the foetus and the neonate. Metabolism of compounds when compared with older animals may be considerably different.

BUTLER. Dr. ROE, you mention non-carcinogens increasing the incidence of tumours. What do you mean by this?

ROE. There are compounds, 3-aminochrysine for example, for which the only evidence of carcinogenicity is this increase in tumour incidence in mice, even after testing in other species.

HOLLANDER. You mention in your paper that the nodules are undoubtedly neoplasms and many are obviously malignant. What criteria do you use? The purpose of this meeting is how to decide this. Two views have been expressed: *(1)* only those lesions which have metastasised and invade are malignant, and *(2)* using morphology and experience, neoplasia and malignant neoplasia can be diagnosed without metastases. If the first view is taken, much of the published work on chemical carcinogenesis would be discarded. I favour the latter view, not just because of the caution in testing, but because we must quantify our data. These problems must be kept in mind at present but at the moment I can offer no solution. I would consider that you can use the mouse for studying mechanisms but am less happy about its use in testing.

142

ROE. I would consider those lesions with metastases, emboli and invasion as malignant neoplasms and the non-metastasising nodules as benign neoplasms.

P. M. NEWBERNE. If you have a 50% incidence in the controls of a neoplasm and this is increased to 100% following treatment, what does this mean? In your Fig. 3 the compound moves the curve to the left. Can this be considered induction of carcinoma? This type of information is often used to demonstrate that the compound is carcinogenic but can it be accepted as evidence of this?

ROE. I think you have pointed directly at the nub of the problem. In the circumstances you have described in your question I believe it would be ridiculous to assume that such an observation indicated that the compound in question is a carcinogen in the sense that it transformed normal cells to cancer cells and thereby *induced* cancer. On the other hand, it is possible to argue that all carcinogens may act simply by increasing the incidence of spontaneously occurring neoplasms *i.e.* by moving the incidence curve to the left. If this is so then there is no fundamental difference between the effect of increasing the life-time incidence of a neoplasm from, say, 0.1% to 50% or from 50% to 100% as in your example. In any event common sense dictates that the first of these situations is far more worrying than the second in relation to the prediction of possible risk for man especially if the 50 to 100% rise can be brought about non-specifically merely by altering food intake or by other means.

THORPE. I would not consider this to be evidence of carcinogenicity. If the compound stimulated the appetite, increasing food intake, this can increase the incidence of neoplasia. I would then not necessarily consider the compound to be a carcinogen.

Chapter 8

Transplantation Studies

Part A—M. D. REUBER*

Part B—J. B. M. GELLATLY

Part A

MELVIN D. REUBER

11014 Swansfield Road, Columbia, Md. 21044 (U.S.A.)

The ultimate criteria for malignancy are the spread of carcinomas by invasion in the liver, extension into nearby organs or metastases to other organs by blood stream or lymphatics. Since such data are not available and may not become available another means of evaluation must be provided. The most reliable method is the subcutaneous transplantation of a fragment of tissue to an untreated isologous host using inbred animals of the same strain. Transplantation studies make possible a correlation of the biologic behaviour with the histological pattern of tumours. Furthermore, the results can be used for interpretation of tumours in random-bred animals (Reuber, 1974).

The first attempts at transplanting tumours of the liver in mice utilized hyperplastic nodules or well-differentiated hepatocellular carcinomas either of unknown origin (EDWARDS *et al.*, 1942b; LEDUC, 1959; REUBER, 1971, ANDERVONT AND DUNN, 1952; LEDUC AND WILSON, 1963; LEDUC *et al.*, 1974) or induced by carbon tetrachloride, 4-*O*-tolylazo-*O*-toluidine or *o*-aminoazotoluene (ANDERVONT AND DUNN, 1952, 1955; LEDUC AND WILSON, 1959; SATO *et al.*, 1956). Not unexpectedly most did not grow on transplantation. More recently poorly differentiated carcinomas, as well as sarcomas, of the liver have been induced in mice by ethylnitrosourea which are readily transplantable (KYRIAZIS AND VESSELINOVITCH, 1973).

Hyperplastic nodules and carcinomas of unknown origin in the livers of untreated mice have been studied in order to correlate the morphological with the biological behaviour of these lesions (REUBER, 1971). This study used C3H × Y hybrid mice in which there are not only a larger number of hepatic lesions, but the lesions develop early in the life of the mouse (HESTON AND VLAHAKIS, 1961; HESTON *et al.*, 1966; HESTON, 1966; VLAHAKIS AND HESTON, 1971). In addition, histological sections from

*Editor's note. This paper has been taken in part from the submitted manuscript and in part from the recordings of the workshop.

transplant studies done by ANDERVONT with liver tumours from mice given carbon tetrachloride, *o*-aminoazotoluene, dieldrin or aldrin, as well as from mice not given chemicals, and from transplant studies done by G. VLAHAKIS (WOODS AND VLAHAKIS, 1973) have been studied.

Most of the work to be described utilized weanling or adult mice as recipients for transplants. However, two well-differentiated hepatocellular carcinomas developing in mice ingesting DDT grew in newborn mice and not adults (TOMATIS *et al.*, 1972).

Hepatic neoplasms can be classified as being either hepatocellular or cholangiocellular in origin. In both instances in poorly differentiated carcinomas the histological criteria for diagnosis are those of anaplasia and one does not have problems of diagnosis. These lesions metastasize most frequently. The problems arise in deciding whether a hepatocellular lesion is a well-differentiated carcinoma or hyperplastic nodule. The same confusion may arise with cholangiocellular neoplasia but we do not have many lesions of this type in mice to study.

All well differentiated carcinomas 1 cm or larger in size in my laboratory grow on transplantation retaining many of the characteristics of normal liver cells and grow in cords two to several cells in thickness (Fig. 1). Sinusoids, with lining cells, may vary from inconspicuous to large and dilated. The cells vary in size and shape with a darkly eosinophilic cytoplasm (Fig. 2). The nuclei are vesicular with a prominent nucleolus. Poorly differentiated hepatocellular carcinomas grow in sheets. The cells vary in size and shape and attempt to form canaliculae. The cytoplasm is basophilic and usually decreased.

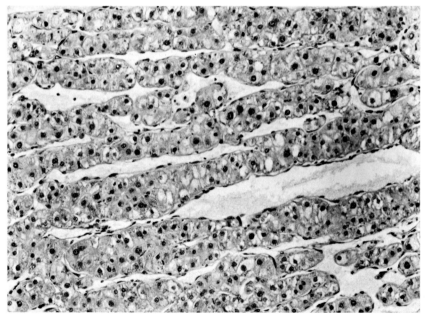

Fig. 1. Well-differentiated hepatocellular carcinoma. Cells are growing in broad cords with wide spaces separating them. Cytoplasm of some cells contain water and/or lipid. Lining cells are conspicuous. Haematoxylin and eosin. ×150.

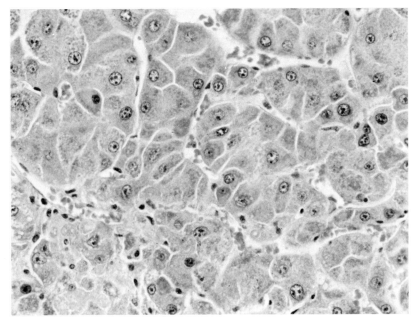

Fig. 2. Moderately well differentiated hepatocellular carcinoma. Nuclei are vesicular with prominent nucleoli. Abundant cytoplasm is eosinophilic. There are lining cells. Haematoxylin and eosin. × 350.

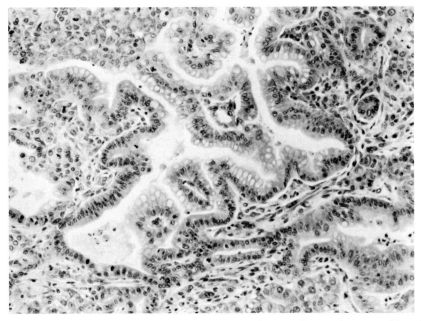

Fig. 3. Well-differentiated cholangiocellular carcinoma. Carcinoma cells are columnar and have basal pseudostratified nuclei with eosinophilic cytoplasm. Clear mucin vacuoles are seen in the apical regions. There are papillary projections into the lumen of the duct. "Desmoplastic" connective tissue stroma is present in the background. Haematoxylin and eosin. ×224.

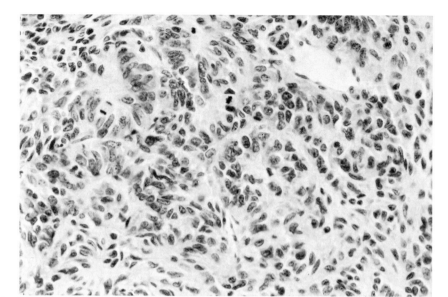

Fig. 4. Poorly differentiated cholangiocellular carcinoma. Cells grow in sheets and attempt to form ducts in some parts. Fibrous connective tissue is present in the background. Haematoxylin and eosin. ×350.

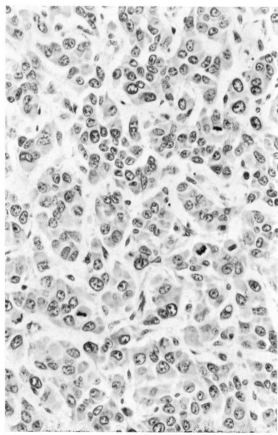

Fig. 5. Undifferentiated carcinoma. Nuclei vary in size and shape. Some are round and others oval. Haematoxylin and eosin. ×350.

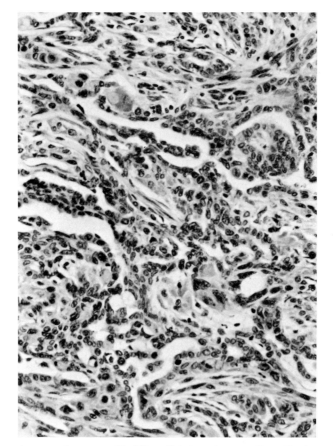

Fig. 6. Mixed carcinoma and sarcoma. Undifferentiated carcinoma cells are lined up and appear to be forming ducts. Spindle-shaped sarcoma cells are also present. Haematoxylin and eosin. ×272.

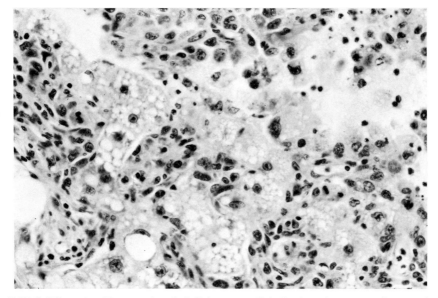

Fig. 7. Well-differentiated haemangioendothelial sarcoma. Spindle-shaped sarcoma cells are replacing the sinusoids. Nuclei are oval and cytoplasm is lightly basophilic. Remaining carcinoma cells have degenerating lipid vacuoles or water in the cytoplasm. Haematoxylin and eosin. ×224.

Cholangiocellular carcinomas retain many of the characteristics of bile duct cells with basophilic columnar epithelium (Fig. 3). In the poorly differentiated form, the neoplasm grows in sheets with a fibrous stroma (Fig. 4). Cholangiocellular carcinomas may be mixed with hepatocellular carcinomas. Undifferentiated carcinomas grow in sheets (Figs. 5 and 6) and are more anaplastic than the poorly differentiated carcinomas. Haemangioendothelial sarcomas (Fig. 7) have also been successfully transplanted.

Hyperplastic nodules grow in sheets with a similar appearance throughout the nodule. The appearance of solid sheets is attributable to the collapse of the sinusoids. When a malignant change occurs, it is first recognized by dilated sinusoids and usually occurs in the centre of the nodule.

Therefore in the absence of metastases there is transplantation which will give additional information. If the tissue grows and survives, the lesion is malignant and if it does not grow it is not malignant. There are several sites for transplantation, the best being intrahepatic particularly if one wishes to study the ability of the transplant to metastasize. In addition intramuscular, subcutaneous, intraperitoneal and intrasplenic routes have been used. Rat tumours have been transplanted to all of these sites with success. However, to study such parameters as growth rate, it is important to be able to observe and palpate the tumour, *i.e.* subcutaneously.

The ultrastructure of transplantable mouse hepatocellular carcinomas retain some of the characteristics of hepatocytes. They have typical nuclei, mitochondria, glycogen, lysosomes, bile canaliculi, Golgi complexes and microbodies. The cisternae of the endoplasmic reticulum are usually simplified but show considerable variation. There is reported to be little correlation between the ultrastructure and the rate of growth. No viruses were reported (TROTTER, 1963; MALICH, 1972). Eosinophilic cytoplasmic inclusion bodies containing protein, which are often seen in primary tumours, are present in transplanted hepatomas during the first generation transplant, but are not usually found in later generations (LEIBELT *et al.*, 1971).

There is a wide range in the growth rate of carcinomas which tends to increase in subsequent generations (HEAD AND LAIRD, 1961; REUBER, 1971). AKAMATSU *et al.* (1969) reported an initial survival time of 13–25 weeks for the 9th generation. Similarly KYRIAZIS AND VESSELINOVITCH (1973) report an initial generation time of 8·4–10·7 weeks which upon subsequent transplantation reduced to about 2 weeks.

Metastases from transplanted tumours are rarely seen, however ALBERT AND ORLOWSKY (1960a) reported a 55% incidence in multiple generations of a tumour originally induced by chrysoidin. KYRIAZIS AND VESSELINOVITCH (1973) also reported lymph node and lung metastases from the second generation. SATO *et al.*, (1956) reported that less well-differentiated carcinomas induced by carbon tetrachloride and 4-O-tolylazo-O-toluidine could be converted into the ascites from an intraperitoneal transplantation and that well-differentiated carcinomas could not.

Some transplanted tumours have polyploid chromosomes, which is consistent with the ploidy of a large number of hepatocytes in the mouse liver (LEDUC *et al.*, 1974). However, neither ploidy nor number and kind of marker chromosomes could be correlated with the histology.

A circadian rhythm in the mitotic activity for a slow and a fast growing transplanted hepatoma has been reported by LLANOS AND NASH (1970). Higher mitotic rates were observed in both during light periods than in dark periods. The fast growing SS1K hepatoma presented consistently higher figures than the slow growing SS1H hepatoma during the dark period while in the light period no significant difference was seen. Thus the variation was greater in the slow growing hepatomas and approached that of immature mouse liver. The finding of change in the mitotic index correlated with the circadian rhythm for DNA synthesis (NASH AND LLANOS, 1971). TROTTER (1961) studied the effect of partial hepatectomy on the mitotic index of transplanted hepatomas and failed to find any significant increased rate in tumours measuring 1 cm diam. However, she reported that on initial transplantation the tumour appeared earlier in animals with partial hepatectomy. This effect was lost in subsequent generations.

The growth of transplanted mouse hepatocellular carcinomas may be altered by a variety of procedures. Irradiation, castration of male mice, partial hepatectomy and splenectomy significantly shortened the latent period of a transplantable chrysoidin carcinoma. The transplants also were rejected more frequently in the animals with intact spleens (SZEWOZUK AND ALBERT, 1973). Anti-lymphocyte serum alone or in combination with either or both prednisone and azothioprine gave a marked increase in the average acceptance rates of a transplanted mouse hepatoma 129. Anti-lymphocyte serum together with azothioprine produced the most consistent and largest increases (PREJEAN et al., 1972).

Biochemical studies have been carried out, often with the intention of correlating the findings with the growth rate or histologic pattern. ALBERT AND ORLOWSKY (1960b) demonstrated an increased oxygen consumption and a normal rate of aerobic glycolysis compared with normal mouse liver and a greatly increased rate of anaerobic glycolysis. Similar findings are reported by WOODS AND VLAHAKIS (1973). The same transplanted hepatoma had a normal level of glucose-6-phosphate dehydrogenase (ALBERT AND ORLOWSKY, 1960c). AKAMATSU et al. (1969) reported that the levels of glucose-6-phosphatase, ATPase, cytochrome b_5 and cytochrome P-450 were similar to normal liver or slightly reduced. Further it was reported that aniline hydroxylation was reduced by one half. HANCOCK AND GRUNAU (1970) studied the soluble ribonucleic acid (sRNA) methylase activity and found variable amounts which did not correlate with rate of growth. REYNOLDS et al. (1971) also studied the enzyme activities of transplantable mouse hepatomas.

DISCUSSION

Pathologists and biologists working and studying spontaneous or induced lesions of the liver in C3H, C3H × Y hybrid, and other strains of mice often have not distinguished between hyperplasia and neoplasia. ANDERVONT AND DUNN (1955) concluded that all lesions of the liver regardless of size or morphology were neoplastic, and that there was no correlation between the transplantability and the morphologic pattern of hepatic lesions. LEMON (1967) and others felt that it was difficult to distinguish between benign and malignant liver tumours in mice and suggested the terminology that liver tumours were "hepatomas" unless metastases were present in which case the lesions were called "carcinomas".

It is important that any tissue taken for transplantation should be carefully selected. It is not unusual for hyperplastic nodules and carcinomas in the same liver to collide and on gross appearance to appear as one large lesion (Fig. 8). If the transplanted tissue and that taken for histological examination were chosen at random, neither would be representative of the tissue transplant. It is necessary to carefully select a lesion and take tissue for transplantation and for histological study from immediately

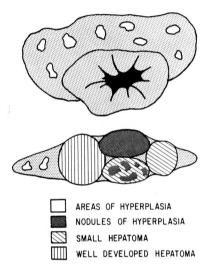

☐ AREAS OF HYPERPLASIA
▨ NODULES OF HYPERPLASIA
▨ SMALL HEPATOMA
▥ WELL DEVELOPED HEPATOMA

Fig. 8. Collision of lesions in the liver. Externally the lesion appears to be a solitary tumour (above). On the cut surface this tumour is made up of four separate lesions (below) (REUBER, 1966).

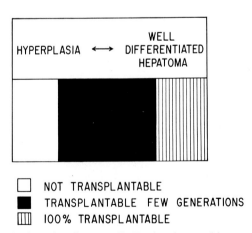

☐ NOT TRANSPLANTABLE
■ TRANSPLANTABLE FEW GENERATIONS
▥ 100% TRANSPLANTABLE

Fig. 9. Mixture of hyperplastic and malignant cells. During the transition stage there are both hyperplastic cells and malignant cells (shown in black) present in the same lesion (REUBER, 1966).

adjacent areas. Tissue taken from nodules showing the transition stage from hyper-plasia to carcinomas may be difficult to transplant and when successful may grow for only one generation. However, tissue from well developed carcinomas can be easily transplanted (REUBER AND FIRMINGER, 1963; REUBER, 1971) (Fig. 9).

Lesions in untreated mice are usually hyperplastic nodules, but some are well differentiated hepatocellular carcinomas (REUBER, 1971). The nodules induced by either carbon tetrachloride or o-aminoazotoluene histologically often resembled hyperplastic lesions rather than carcinomas and as reported by ANDERVONT AND DUNN (1952) do not transplant. The undifferentiated carcinomas induced by ethyl-nitrosourea are readily transplantable, metastasize widely and kill the host (KYRIAZIS AND VESSELINOVITCH, 1973). The results of transplantation of hepatic lesions in mice are similar to those lesions in rats induced by chemical carcinogens (REUBER, 1963, 1966). Hyperplastic lesions will not grow whereas carcinomas will grow on trans-plantation. (REUBER AND FIRMINGER, 1963; REUBER, 1966, 1971; REUBER AND ODASHIMA, 1967). However, metastases of primary and transplantable well differen-tiated hepatocellular carcinomas in rats kill the host more often than in mice.

Neoplasms derived from the non-parenchymal cell tissue are also transplantable. TOMATIS et al. (1972) observed poorly differentiated cholangiocarcinomas in mice receiving DDT. While transplantation studies were not done, similar cholangiocar-cinomas have been transplanted by REUBER (1971) and WOODS AND VLAHAKIS (1973). TRAININ (1963) successfully transplanted well-differentiated haemangioendo-thelial sarcomas which had been induced with urethane. A similar spontaneous trans-plantable well-differentiated haemangioendothelial sarcoma has been transplanted (EDWARDS et al., 1942a). Leiomyosarcomas and reticulum cell sarcomas of the liver have been successfully transplanted from mice ingesting dieldrin and aldrin.

ANDERVONT AND DUNN (1952, 1955) reported that hepatic carcinomas in mice developed into haemangiosarcomas, fibrosarcomas, reticulum cell sarcomas and adenocarcinomas on successive transplantations. The likely explanation for this observation is that more than one lesion was transplanted and later the more malignant lesion, i.e. the sarcoma, outgrew the less malignant well-differentiated hepatocellular carcinomas. It is not unusual for mixed hepatic tumours to develop in the mouse liver, and for these to grow on transplantation.

SUMMARY

Carcinomas and sarcomas of the liver occurring in mice can readily be transplanted. There is a close correlation between the morphologic and biologic behaviour of the transplanted carcinomas which grossly and histologically resemble the primary transplanted tumour. The better differentiated carcinomas grow slowly, however, the poorly and undifferentiated carcinomas grow rapidly. Transplantable carcinomas often retain characteristics of normal hepatocytes as shown by ultrastructural and biochemical studies.

REFERENCES

AKAMATSU, Y., WADA, F., AND IKEGAMI, R. (1969) Transplantation of spontaneous hepatomas in C3H mice: Biological and biochemichal studies. *Gann*, 60: 145.

ALBERT, Z., AND ORLOWSKY, M. (1960a) Some peculiar biological and biochemical properties of a mouse hepatoma induced by chrysoidin, I. Biological and biochemical characteristics of the hepatoma. *J. Natl. Cancer Inst.*, 25: 443.

ALBERT, Z., AND ORLOWSKY, M. (1960b) Some peculiar biological and biochemical properties of a mouse hepatoma induced by chrysoidin, II. Metabolic properties of a mouse hepatoma induced by chrysoidin, II. Metabolic properties of the hepatoma. *J. Natl. Cancer Inst.*, 25: 455.

ALBERT, Z., AND ORLOWSKY, M. (1960c) Some peculiar biological and biochemical properties of a mouse hepatoma induced by chrysoidi 1, III. Activity of glucose-6-phosphatase. *J. Natl. Cancer Inst.*, 25: 461.

ANDERVONT, H. B., AND DUNN, T. B. (1952) Transplantation of spontaneous and induced hepatomas in inbred mice. *J. Natl. Cancer Inst.*, 13: 455.

ANDERVONT, H. B. AND DUNN, T. B. (1955) Transplantation of hepatomas in mice. *J. Natl. Cancer Inst., Suppl.*, 15: 1513.

EDWARDS, J. E., ANDERVONT, H. B., AND DALTON, A. (1942a) A transplantable malignant hemangio-endothelioma of the liver in the mouse. *J. Natl. Cancer Inst.*, 2: 479.

EDWARDS, J. E., DALTON, A. J., AND ANDERVONT, H. B. (1942b) Pathology of transplantable sponta-neous hepatoma in a C3H mouse. *J. Natl. Cancer Inst.*, 2: 555.

HANCOCK, R. L., AND GRUNAU, J. (1970) Soluble RNA methylase activity of transplantable mouse hepatoma. *J. Natl. Cancer Inst.*, 45: 971.

HEAD, M. A., AND LAIRD, H. M. (1961) A histological study of the latent period of hepatoma grafts. *Brit J. Cancer*, 15: 615.

HESTON, W. E. (1966) Factors in the causation of spontaneous hepatomas in mice. *J. Natl. Cancer Inst.*, 37: 839.

HESTON, W. E., AND VLAHAKIS, G. (1961) Influence of the A^y gene on mammary-gland tumors, hepatomas, and normal growth in mice. *J. Natl. Cancer Inst.*, 26: 969.

HESTON, W. E., VLAHAKIS, G., AND DERINGER, M. K. (1966) High incidence of spontaneous hepatomas and the increase of this incidence with urethan in C3H, C3Hf and C3He male mice. *J. Natl. Cancer Inst.*, 24: 425.

KYRIAZIS, A. P., AND VESSELINOVITCH, S. D. (1973) Transplantability and biological behavior of mouse liver tumors. *Cancer Res.*, 33: 332.

LEDUC, E. H. (1959) Metastasis of transplantable hepatomas from the spleen to the liver in mice. *Cancer Res.*, 19: 1091.

LEDUC, E. H. AND WILSON, J. W. (1959) Transplantation of carbon tetrachloride-induced hepatomas in mice. *J. Natl. Cancer Inst.*, 22: 581.

LEDUC, E. H., AND WILSON, J. W. (1963) Production of transplantable hepatomas by intrasplenic implantation of normal liver in mouse. *J. Natl. Cancer Inst.*, 30: 85.

LEDUC, E. H. MALICK, L. E., AND HOLDEN, H. E. (1974) Light microscopic observations of trans-plantable mouse hepatomas. *Cancer Res.*, 34: 716.

LEMON, P. G. (1967) Hepatic neoplasms of rats and mice. In: *Pathology of Laboratory Rats and Mice*, Chapter 2, pp. 25–56. COTCHIN, F., AND ROE, J. C. R., (Eds.) Blackwell, Oxford.

LIEBELT, A. G., LIEBELT, R. A., AND DMOCHOWSKY, L. (1971) Cytoplasmic inclusion bodies in primary and transplanted hepatomas of mice of different strains. *J. Natl. Cancer Inst.*, 47: 413.

LLANOS, J. M., AND NASH, R. E. (1970) Mitotic circadian rhythm in a fast-growing and a slow-grow-ing hepatoma. Mitotic rhythm in hepatoma. *J. Natl. Cancer Inst.*, 44: 581.

MALICK, L. E. (1972) Ultrastructure of transplantable mouse hepatomas of different rates. *J. Natl. Cancer Inst.*, 49: 1033.

NASH, R. E., AND LLANOS, J. M. (1971) Twenty-four-hour variations in DNA synthesis of a fast-growing and a slow growing hepatoma. *J. Natl. Cancer Inst.*, 47: 1007.

PREJEAN, J. D., GRISWOLD, D. P., AND WEISBURGER, J. H. (1972) Transplantation of allogenic tumors in rats and mice treated with azathioprine, prednisone and antilymphocyte serum. *Proc. Soc. Exp. Biol. Med.*, 139: 1425.

REUBER, M. D. (1966) Histopathology of transplantable hepatic carcinomas induced by chemical carcinogens in rats. *Gann Monograph*, 1: 43.

REUBER, M. D. (1967) Poorly differentiated cholangiocarcinomas occurring "spontaneously" in C3H and C3H × Y hybrid mice. *J. Natl. Cancer Inst.*, 38: 901.

REUBER, M. D. (1971) Morphologic and biologic correlation of hyperplastic and neoplastic hepatic lesions occurring "spontaneously" in C3H × Y hybrid mice, *Brit. J. Cancer*, 25: 538.

REUBER, M. D., AND FIRMINGER, H. I. (1963) Morphologic and biologic correlation of liver lesions obtained in hepatic carcinogenesis in A × C rats given 0·025 per cent N,2-fluorenyldiacetamide. *J. Natl. Cancer Inst.*, 31: 1407.

REUBER, M. D., AND ODASHIMA, S. (1967) Further studies on the transplantation of lesions in hepatic carcinogenesis in rats given 2-(diacetoamido)fluorene, *Gann*, 58: 513.

REUBER, M. D. (1974) Criteria for tumor diagnosis and classification of malignancy. In: *Carcinogenesis Testing of Chemicals*, pp. 71–73.

GOLBERG, L. (Ed.), CRC Press, Cleveland, Ohio.

REYNOLDS, R. D., POTTER, V. R., PITOT, H. C., AND REUBER, M. D. (1971) Survey of some enzyme patterns in transplantable Reuber mouse hepatomas, *Cancer Res.*, 31: 808.

SATO, H., BELKIN, M., AND ESSNER, E. (1956) Experiments on an ascites hepatoma, III. The conversion of mouse hepatomas into the ascites form. *J. Natl. Cancer Inst.*, 17: 1.

SZEWOZUK, A., AND ALBERT, Z. (1973) Activity of some hydroloses in animals with transplanted and spontaneous tumours. *Folia Histochem. Cytochem.*, 11: 73.

TOMATIS, L., TURUSOV, V., DAY, N., AND CHARLES, R. T. (1972) The effect of long-term exposure to DDT on F-1 mice. *Int. J. Cancer*, 10: 489.

TRAININ, N. (1963) Neoplastic nature of liver "blood cysts" induced by urethane in mice. *J. Natl. Cancer Inst.*, 31: 1489.

TROTTER, N. L. (1961) The effect of partial hepatectomy on subcutaneous transplanted hepatoma in mice. *Cancer Res.*, 21: 778.

TROTTER, N. L. (1963) Electron microscopic observations on cytoplasmic components of transplantable hepatomas in mice. *J. Natl. Cancer Inst.*, 30: 113.

VLAHAKIS, G., AND HESTON, W. E. (1971) Spontaneous cholangioma in strain C3H A^{vy}fB mice and their hybrids. *J. Natl. Cancer Inst.*, 46: 677.

WOODS, M. W., AND VLAHAKIS, G. (1973) Anaerobic glycolysis in spontaneous and transplanted liver tumors of mice. *J. Natl. Cancer Inst.*, 50: 1497.

Part B

J. B. M. GELLATLY

Unilever Research Laboratory, Colworth House, Sharnbrook, Bedford (Great Britain)

INTRODUCTION

Since many workers including EDWARDS *et al.* (1942), ANDERVONT AND DUNN (1952), TAPER *et al.*, (1966), AKAMATSU *et al.*, (1969) and REUBER (1971) have demonstrated the transplantability of spontaneous hepatomas in mice and since it was considered that this technique might prove of value in differentiating nodules of hyperplasia from those in which neoplastic transformation had occurred, a small-scale transplantation study was undertaken in this laboratory (FERRIGAN *et al.*, unpublished observations). Although the Colworth C57BL mouse is highly inbred, determination of genetic similarity among randomly selected individuals was considered necessary, prior to transplantation studies of hepatic nodules. This was accomplished by the grafting of donor, hairless, aural skin to the backs of the recipients. Such grafts survived for an indefinite period, thus demonstrating their isograft nature.

METHODS

Hepatic nodules, used for transplantation, were obtained from mice killed at the termination of 80-week trials and varied in size from 2–20 mm in diameter; nodules showing extensive necrosis/haemorrhage on their cut surface were not selected, since survival of such lesions was considered unlikely. One half of each selected nodule was fixed in 10% formol saline for subsequent histological examination; the other half was placed in isotonic saline, cut into 1–2 mm cubes as soon as possible and transplanted within 30 min of the donor's death. Recipient mice (4–8 per nodule) were 8 weeks old and of both sexes. The kidney (subcapsular intrarenal site) was selected for transplantation since, although a heterotopic site, macroscopic and histological differentiation between hepatic graft and host tissue is much easier in this site than in the orthotopic site. Furthermore, the renal capsule holds the grafts securely until established or rejected. Following laparotomy, a portion of a selected hepatic nodule was inserted beneath the left renal capsule and a portion of normal hepatic tissue, from the same animal, was similarly located in the right kidney. Three months later, gross inspection of the grafts was made following laparotomy.

In addition to grafts of hepatic nodules, grafts were also made of portions of liver from mice at periods of maximum physiological, hepatic mitotic activity. Since WILSON *et al.* (1970) had demonstrated, during a study of physiological hepatic enlargement during pregnancy and lactation in the rat, that peak mitotic activity was attained around the 14th day of pregnancy and the 14th day of lactation, grafts of mouse liver, obtained at similar stages of pregnancy and lactation, were also transplanted. Likewise, since mitotic activity is high in newborn mouse liver, transplantation studies of this tissue were undertaken. Heterograft studies were also made, in the course of which portions of normal liver and of parenchymal nodules were transplanted to the cheek pouch of the Syrian hamster.

This study was undertaken in two parts; in the first, the recipient mice were killed after 6–10 weeks in order to assess the viability and growth potential of grafted tissue from moderate to large-sized parenchymal nodules. In the second, recipients were allowed to survive for one year from receipt of transplants taken from parenchymal nodules of all sizes. During these studies, all recipient mice were fed stock pelleted diet *ad lib.*

RESULTS

Short-term study

Hepatic parenchymal nodules selected for this study varied in size from 7–15 mm diameter; smaller nodules were not used, since the primary objective was assessment of the ability of transplants to become established in the recipient kidney and it was considered more likely that this could be achieved by grafts of larger nodules.

Portions of 11 nodules from untreated C57BL mice of 86–88 weeks of age were transplanted into 45 recipient mice; 24 isografts from 8 donor nodules were found to be viable 6–10 weeks after implantation. Many of these transplants showed morphological characteristics of the original nodule, *e.g.* nuclear enlargement, intranuclear and intracytoplasmic inclusions, intense cytoplasmic basophilia, *etc.* One feature observed in 17 of the 24 established isografts, *viz.* "oval" cell proliferation, frequently simulating biliary epithelial hyperplasia, was not present in the original nodules. Of the 8 donor nodules which provided viable transplants, six were of Type 2 and two were of Type 3 in the classification system adopted in Chapter 5; two of the three nodules which failed to produce viable transplants were of Type 1 and the third was of Type 2.

This study not only demonstrated the feasibility of intrarenal transplantation of hepatic parenchymal nodules in Colworth C57BL mice but also suggested that nodules of certain morphological types were more liable to become established than others. It was also observed that donor tissue from males or females had a greater tendency to become established in recipients of the same sex. On the basis of these results, a one-year study of transplants from nodules of all sizes was undertaken.

One-year study

Hepatic parenchymal nodules selected for this study varied in size from 2–20 mm diameter; 11 nodules were used for transplantation of which 5 were of 2–4 mm diameter and 6 of 5–20 mm diameter. All nodules were obtained from untreated C57BL mice killed at 86–88 weeks of age and portions of these 11 lesions were transplanted into the kidneys of 64 recipients. Three months after transplantation, laparotomy was performed on each recipient and both kidneys were examined for evidence of transplant growth. At this time, intrarenal foci were identified in 16 recipients of tissue from 5 donor hepatic nodules; 11 of the renal lesions were approx. 1 mm diameter but 5 (all from the same donor nodule, 1536) were 4–6 mm diameter.

During the next 9 months, 12 of the original 64 recipients died or were killed due to ill health. In 6 of these animals, nodules varying in size from 15–40 mm were detected in the left kidney; 5 of these 6 mice had received isografts from the same donor (1536) and in all 5 cases, it was considered that the terminal illness of the animal, 5–8 months after transplantation, was due to growth of a transplanted neoplasm. All 52 surviving recipients were killed one year after the initial transplant operation. At necropsy, nodules of 10–30 mm diameter were detected in 11 recipients of tissue from 4 donor nodules. Thus, of the original 64 recipients of tissue from 11 nodules, isograft growth developed in 17 from 5 donor nodules. Of the 5 donor nodules which provided viable transplants, 3 were of Type 2 and 2 were of Type 3 in our classification system while, of the 6 nodules which did not grow in the recipient kidneys, 4 were of Type 1 and 2 of Type 2.

Several features of interest were noted during this study, one of the most interesting being the rapid growth of isografts from donor 1536 and the malignant characteristics

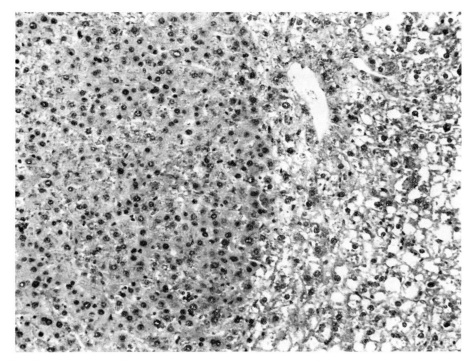

Fig. 10. Transplantable Type 2 nodule composed almost exclusively of small basophil cells: mouse fed purified diet (10·0% groundnut oil). Compare intrarenal transplant, Fig. 11). H.P.S. × 180.

158

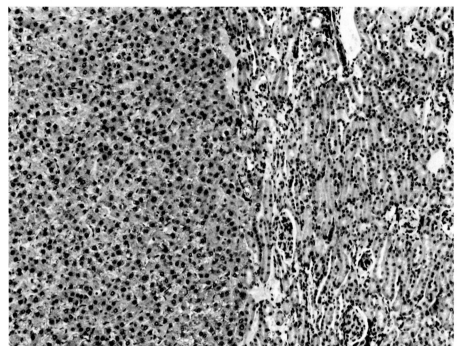

Fig. 11. Expansive growth of intrarenal transplant of Type 2 nodule (Fig. 1), 1 year after implantatin. H.P.S. × 135.

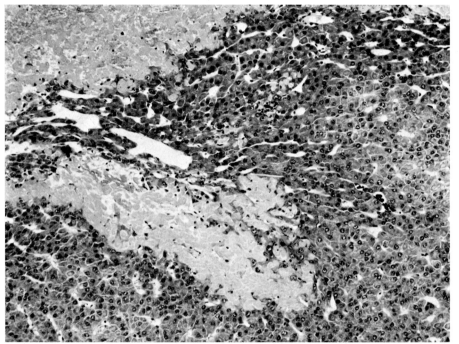

Fig. 12. Invasive growth and necrosis in intrarenal transplant of Type 3 nodule: implant growth totally replaced kidney and metastasized throughout abdomen, killing animal 6 months after implantation. H.P.S. ×135.

of renal invasion, poor differentiation and transcoelomic metastases exhibited by these transplants. This finding is of particular importance since the donor nodule was one of the few in our series which contained areas resembling the poorly differentiated hepatoblastoma described by TURUSOV *et al.* (1973). A second feature of interest was the influence of the sex of the recipients on establishment of transplants. Thus, of 17 established transplants, 14 occurred in recipients of the same sex as the donor and only 3 in the opposite sex; of these latter three, two were mice which had been implanted with the highly malignant neoplasm from donor 1536. Overall, establishment and growth in male recipients appeared to be better than in females.

Histological studies of these intrarenal transplants revealed a variable degree of similarity between the morphology of the donor nodule (Fig. 10) and that of the isografts (Fig. 11). In two cases, the dominant morphological features of the original nodule were closely replicated. In one (1536), both donor nodule (Type 3) and recipient isografts demonstrated a poorly differentiated hepatocellular carcinoma which, in the recipient, invaded the kidney and metastasized widely throughout the abdomen (Fig. 12). In the other, a well-differentiated Type 2 donor nodule, a high degree of uniform differentiation was maintained in the isograft with evidence of only expansive growth in the kidney. The other three donor nodules which provided viable transplants were all of a complex type with widely differing morphological patterns intermingled within them, *e.g.* solid and trabecular structure, small and large cells, acidophil and basophil cells, areas rich in intracytoplasmic inclusions. In the isografts, similar

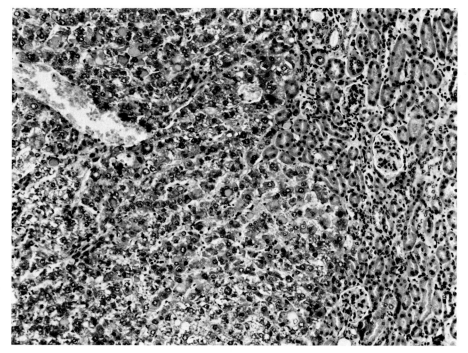

Fig. 13. Expansive growth of intrarenal transplant of Type 2 nodule, containing numerous acidophil intracytoplasmic inclusions, 1 year after implantation. H.P.S. ×135.

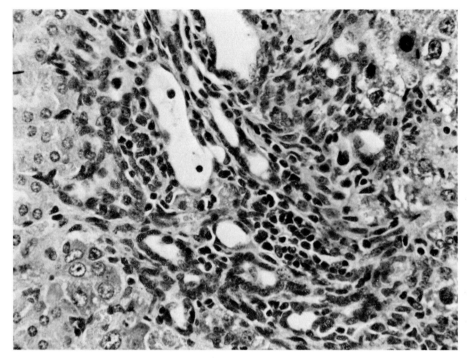

Fig. 14. "Oval" cell proliferation and ductule formation in intrarenal transplant of Type 3 nodule (10 weeks after implantation). H.P.S. ×470.

variations were found, but in each, one particular morphological pattern tended to become predominant; thus, the transplants from nodule 1590 (Type 2) were composed of very large cells, with marked nuclear polyploidy and numerous intracytoplasmic inclusions (Fig. 13). The apparent dominance of one pattern in the transplants is possibly a reflection of the area of the original nodule selected for transplantation. One striking feature of over half the transplants was the occurrence of "oval" cell proliferation (Fig. 14). This feature was never conspicuous in the original donor nodules. In the earlier short-term study, structures resembling bile ducts were often associated with this proliferative change but in isografts from the one year study, structures resembling bile ducts were rarely observed; instead, "oval" cell proliferation appeared to be closely associated with the formation of strands of new connective tissue which demarcated ill-defined lobules within the transplant.

DISCUSSION

In general, this study confirmed the observations of ANDERVONT AND DUNN (1952) and AKAMATSU et al. (1969) that the growth of established transplants of hepatic nodules in mice is slow. In the present study, isografts of 4 of the 5 donor nodules grew slowly during the first 12 weeks after transplantation and reached diameters of 10–30 mm after one year. In contrast, however, isografts from nodule 1536 attained sizes of 4–6 mm after 12 weeks and proved fatal 5–8 months after transplantation (15–40 mm diameter).

After one year, grafts taken from pregnant, lactating and newborn mice had totally disappeared, as had implants of "normal" liver. At the sites of transplantation, focal calcification within fibrous scars was identified. All grafts transplanted to the hamster cheek pouches were completely reabsorbed after one month. On histological examination of the kidneys of mice dying or killed due to illness during the first 3 months of the long-term study, regressive changes were observed in grafts of normal liver and grafts from nodules which failed to become established. In none of these cases was there evidence of significant lymphocytic or plasma cell infiltration; the necrobiotic grafts were, however, surrounded and infiltrated by aggregates of polymorphonuclear leucocytes and macrophages. These findings suggest that failure of grafts to become established is not associated with immunological rejection but is influenced by the growth potential of components of individual hepatic parenchymal nodules.

One of the hepatic nodules selected for transplantation proved on histological examination to be a vasoformative neoplasm and on transplantation produced a 10 mm nodule after 1 year. This tumour resembled the transplantable haemangioendothelioma described by ANDERVONT AND DUNN (1952) and AKAMATSU et al. (1967).

Since our transplantation studies were undertaken on a small scale, no attempt will be made to review the literature on this subject. Instead, comment will be restricted to a brief consideration of a few relevant aspects of such studies. As BUTLER (1971) has indicated, transplanted hepatomas may have some advantages as model systems for studying certain features of hepatic parenchymal nodules, e.g. growth rate. The ability to transplant such lesions suggests that they are neoplastic but not necessarily carcinomatous, since transplantation, per se, cannot be considered an absolute indication of malignancy (EDWARDS et al., 1942).

When a hepatic nodule in the original host is compared with isologous transplants in the recipient, one is soon aware, in the majority of cases, of the lack of histological similarity between the two. Transplanted nodules frequently present a much more uniform structure than the original and the dominant cytological features of the transplants are seldom the most characteristic or representative components of the original lesion. In our series, the predominant features of only two donor nodules were replicated in the transplants and in each, the donor nodule was of a type classified by REUBER (1971) as a poorly differentiated or undifferentiated carcinoma. It would appear, therefore, that in the majority of cases, the "impurity" of the cell population within hepatic nodules of mixed morphological character "precludes the application of sophisticated biochemical techniques to an intelligent molecular analysis of a frank malignancy" (MERKOW et al., 1969). It would also appear that serial transplantation of such nodules through many generations, with associated increase in growth rate and further loss of differentiation, must produce a model substantially different in both morphological and behavioural terms from the original lesion with which we are at present concerned.

In our transplantation studies, establishment of isologous transplants was generally more successful in recipients of the same sex as the donor animal. The only exception

162

to this was a hepatocellular carcinoma which, in the donor, had undergone metastases to the lungs and which, in recipients, proved fatal 5–8 months after transplantation. Although the number of transplants undertaken was comparatively small, the influence of sex on successful isograft establishment and/or growth is an interesting one. As pointed out by LIEBELT AND LIEBELT (1967), members of an inbred strain are identical genotypes except for the presence of X and Y chromosomes and isologous grafting of tumours is uniformly successful. The results obtained by EICHWALD AND SILMSER (1955) confirmed by PREHN AND MAIN (1956) have, however, modified this concept since both groups demonstrated that while skin grafts from C57BL male donors to male hosts were almost consistently successful, male grafts were rejected by female hosts, particularly after 6 months when they appeared to be established. The rejection of male grafts has now been observed by numerous investigators using a variety of tissues (LIEBELT AND LIEBELT, 1967) and although rejection has been recorded in many strains, the results of EICHWALD et al. (1958) indicate that the factor is strongest in C57BL mice. The mechanism of male to female rejection is unknown but there is evidence that a transplantation immunity phenomenon, similar to homograft rejection as described by MEDAWAR (1944), is involved and that rejection of male tissue is determined by the presence of one or more autosomal genes which enable females to react to male-specific antigen (EICHWALD AND WETZEL, 1965). No reference to male rejection of female tissue has been found in the literature.

This study demonstrates that a proportion of spontaneous hepatic parenchymal nodules in Colworth C57BL mice are transplantable and that while the majority of established isografts grow slowly by expansion, some are capable of rapid growth with tissue invasion and the production of metastases. It is considered highly significant that while none of the Type 1 nodules transplanted grew in the recipient kidney, all the Type 3 nodules and a proportion of the Type 2 series became established and grew in the intrarenal site. This evidence supports the view that while all of our Type 3 nodules and at least a proportion of our Type 2 are tumours, lesions of Type 1 represent foci of nodular hyperplasia.

ACKNOWLEDGEMENT

In the preparation of this paper, the author has included data from the transplantation studies of Dr. L. FERRIGAN; the use of this material is gratefully acknowledged.

REFERENCES

AKAMATSU, Y., TAKEMURA, T., IKEGAMI, R., TAKAHASHI, A., AND MIYAJIMA, H. (1967) Growth behavior of hepatomas in *o*-aminoazotoluene-treated mice in comparison with spontaneous hepatomas. *Gann*, 58: 323.
AKAMATSU, Y., WADA, F., AND IKEGAMI, R. (1969) Transplantation of spontaneous hepatomas in C3H mice; biological and biochemical studies. *Gann*, 60: 145.
ANDERVONT, H. B., AND DUNN, T. B. (1952) Transplantation of spontaneous and induced hepatomas in inbred mice. *J. Natl. Cancer Inst.*, 13: 455.
BUTLER, W. H. (1971) Pathology of liver cancer in experimental animals. In: *Liver Cancer*, pp. 30–41, I.A.R.C. Scientific Publication No. 1, I.A.R.C., Lyons.

EDWARDS, J. E., DALTON, A. J., AND ANDERVONT, H. B. (1942) Pathology of a transplantable spontaneous hepatoma in a C3H mouse. *J. Natl. Cancer Inst.*, 2: 555.

EICHWALD, E. J., AND SILMSER, C. R. (1955) Communication. *Transplant. Bull.*, 2: 148.

EICHWALD, E. J., AND WETZEL, B. (1965) Rejection of isologous male grafts and the translocation
theory. *Transplantation*, 3: 583.

EICHWALD, E. J., SILMSER, C. R., AND WEISSMAN, I. (1958) Sex-linked rejection of normal and neoplastic tissue, 1. Distribution and specificity. *J. Natl. Cancer Inst.*, 20: 563.

LIEBELT, A. G., AND LIEBELT, R. A. (1967) Transplantation of tumors. In: *Methods in Cancer Research*,
Vol. 1 pp. 143–242. BUSCH, H. (Ed.), Academic Press, London.

MEDAWAR. P. B. (1944) The behaviour and fate of skin autografts and skin homografts in rabbits.
J. Anat., 78: 176.

MERKOW, L. P., EPSTEIN, S. M., FARBER, E., PARDO, M., AND BARTUS, B. (1969) Cellular analysis of
liver carcinogenesis, III. Comparison of the ultrastructure of hyperplastic liver nodules and hepatocellular carcinomas induced in rat liver by 2-fluorenylacetamide. *J. Natl. Cancer Inst.*, 43: 33.

PREHN, R. T., AND MAIN, J. M. (1956) The influence of sex on isologous skin grafting in the mouse.
J. Natl. Cancer Inst., 17: 35.

REUBER, M. D. (1971) Morphologic and biologic correlation of hyperplastic and neoplastic hepatic
lesions occurring "spontaneously" in C3H × Y hybrid mice. *Brit. J. Cancer*, 25: 538.

TAPER, H. S., WOOLLEY, G. W., TELLER, M. N., AND LARDIS, M. P. (1966) A new transplantable
mouse liver tumor of spontaneous origin. *Cancer Res.*, 26: 143.

TURUSOV, V. S., DAY, N. E., TOMATIS, L., GATI, E., AND CHARLES, R. T. (1973) Tumors in CF-1 mice
exposed for six consecutive generations to DDT. *J. Natl. Cancer Inst.*, 51: 983.

WILSON, R., DOELL, B. H., GROGER, W., HOPE, J., AND GELLATLY, J. B. M. (1970) The physiology of
liver enlargement. In: *Metabolic Aspects of Food Safety*, Chapter 15, pp. 363–418. ROE, F. J. C. (Ed.)
Blackwell, Oxford.

DISCUSSION

THORPE. In random-bred strains, if the nodule is transplantable, this is good evidence of autonomous
growth but not evidence of whether it is benign or malignant. Rate of growth and ability to metastasize may give more information of its biological behaviour. With an inbred strain, I am very hesitant
to accept that of itself it is in any way evidence of neoplasia, if the lesion just grows at the site of
transplantation. If metastases can be demonstrated, this may be evidence of neoplasia.

GELLATLY. I would agree with the opinion expressed in the I.A.R.C. Working Conference on Liver
Cancer in that the system may be useful for studying certain features of neoplasia such as growth rate,
but would hesitate to place great significance on it.

GRASSO. I would agree that it may be useful for studying mechanism, but doubt its usefulness as a test
for malignancy.

ROE. Transplantation is obviously difficult to interpret because of false positive and false negative
results, but it may be of value if there is immediate growth. False negatives may result from a number
of factors such as infection, number of viable cells innoculated, blood supply, hormonal and immunological effects. False positives may result from oncogenic viruses and possible tumour progression
after transplantation. In particular, these latter problems arise if the growth is very slow and delayed.

GRICE. I consider that transplantation has no place in routine testing.

TAKAYAMA. Transplantation can be considered evidence of autonomous growth but in order to
diagnose malignancy, requires evidence of invasion or cellular atypism.

REUBER. Everybody finds it easy to dismiss transplantation on theoretical grounds without suggesting
alternatives. The suggestion we have heard as criteria of malignancy, that of invasion and metastases,
are just not practical and would not be acceptable to other people. This group is willing to accept
invasion and metastases in the primary animal in which the carcinoma has the best chance of pro-

gressing to another lesion. However, if one takes it out of the host and places it in another animal and it still grows against all difficulties, this is good evidence of carcinoma.

Roe. Have you ever transplanted a malignant tumour which failed to grow?

Reuber. No, with the qualification that if the tumour is less than 1 cm in diameter it will only grow if transplanted into the liver of another animal, but over 1 cm tumours will transplant into other sites.

Roe. This is not other people's experience who have found that even with undoubted malignant tumours evidence by the presence of metastases that negative results may be obtained. This would be an example of a false negative.

Butler. Do hyperplastic lesions ever transplant?

Reuber. We have one example of this when a lesion diagnosed as hyperplasia grew for only one generation. It had certainly typical features and may be one of those cases of uncertainty of diagnosis.

Roe. It is a common observation in many studies that a transplanted tumour may only grow after a year. I would suggest that this only tells you that the tumour is malignant at the time it grows and not at the time of transplantation. This type of observation tells you nothing of the malignancy at the time of transplantation. If the histological features of the growing tumour fulfill the criteria for malignancy one does not know if it satisfied these criteria at the time of transplantation. This may be an example of tumour progression.

Reuber. In my experience if it takes a year to grow the lesion is unlikely to survive subsequent generations. I think the original host is required for transformation. When a transplant grows for a period and then stops, remaining at the final size, the lesion may be considered hyperplastic although I would like the designation adenoma.

Butler. You use transplantation as a criterion of malignancy and then say that everything that transplants is malignant. This is a circular argument.

Reuber. I am saying that if you transplant many tumours with a certain histological pattern anything that has that pattern is a malignant carcinoma. In those instances with a low incidence of take on transplantation, I presume that there is a mixture of hyperplastic and malignant cells in the original tumour. I do not know how many malignant cells are required for multiple generation transplantation. I follow the same criteria of behaviour and histology in the primary host and the transplant. In some instances a first generation transplant will cease to grow. In this case, I do not consider the lesion to be malignant. A transplant should grow, kill the host and be transplantable over many generations to be considered malignant. If a certain number of primary tumours, carcinomas, of a given histological pattern will invade and metastasize and grow and kill the animal on transplantation the carcinoma is malignant. Following this we can look at slides from any other experiment and indeed I would go further and say in any other species and make the diagnosis of carcinoma on the histological examination alone.

Butler. What views do the group have on the use of inbred strains? Heston has suggested that all work should be done on inbred strains, but others feel that this may be misleading.

J. Newberne. The popularity of inbred strains has been derived from investigators who have studied specific tumour systems by a particular class of compounds. This enthusiasm has been translated to the broad field of testing compounds and I think that there is little use for them in this field. I do not think that I can rely on inbred strains anymore than a random-bred strain. Indeed, I think a better test might be done of an unknown compound if a mouse is used which is not selected for some one particular use.

Reuber. Geneticists use them for obvious reasons and at the National Cancer Institute they have been used extensively in transplantation studies. This usefulness of the transplantation studies required inbred mice as they would not be possible in random-bred mice. If only random-bred mice were used, only highly malignant tumours would be transplantable. It depends on the purpose to which the mice are to be put. If a comparative carcinogenicity test of a series of compounds is to be done, inbred mice would give comparable results and hence be useful. But if an unknown compound is to be tested there are considerable advantages to be derived from the use of more than one set of genes.

Chapter 9

Mouse Hepatic Neoplasia

Significance and Extrapolation to Man

J. W. NEWBERNE

Director, Drug Safety and Metabolism,
Merrell-National Laboratories,
Division of Richardson-Merrell Inc.,
110 E. Amity Road,
Cincinnati, Ohio 45215 (U.S.A.)

When first approached to consider the complex area of the significance of experimental carcinogenicity data and its extrapolation from mouse to man, my first impulse was to suggest that I have great confidence in the ability of future scientists to successfully accomplish this feat and return the meeting to the chairman. Upon further reflection, however, it occurred to me that opportunities to examine this matter and to discuss, debate and perhaps challenge some of the existing dogmas in this regard do not often occur, and that this particular opportunity should not be ignored. Consequently, we will briefly examine this area, and if the opinions of those in attendance will be made known, perhaps some consensus on at least some facets of the problem might be achieved.

In preparing for this workshop, my initial intention was to present an overall review of many relevant factors (*e.g.*, comparative pharmacology, toxicology, metabolism, genetics) concerning which data developed in the mouse and other laboratory species might be collated to help predict potential effects in man. As you know, however, such comparisons have been made many times before, and aside from providing erudite, readable material, and in some cases contributing to the paper shortage, I believe it can be fairly stated that such comparisons have contributed only marginally to our understanding of carcinogenesis. Thus, despite the vast amount of data accumulated from such investigations, as well as our overall experience in defining and comparing biological effects in a variety of animal species, gaps still exist and probably always will in our ability to predict biological effects of compounds across species lines. After digesting the superb review of mouse neoplasia presented at this workshop during the past week, I am now convinced, as I suspect most of you are, that it would be of little value to expound on these rather speculative areas, and my comments have been realigned accordingly.

Before we attempt to extrapolate experimental mouse data to man, we should first deal with a few fundamental questions concerning the mouse liver *per se* which have little, if anything, to do with the broader issue of extrapolating across species lines. These are:

(1) Using all the techniques at our disposal (*e.g.*, morphology, biological behaviour in the host, transplantation, biochemistry, biostatistics), can we develop and define objective criteria for distinguishing between benign and malignant liver nodules in the mouse?

(2) Do agents other than carcinogens induce nodules in the mouse liver?

As has become evident during this workshop, we have been unable to develop a consensus on a precise distinction between benign and malignant neoplasms in the mouse liver, and we have clearly been unable to define objective criteria essential to such judgments. If we accept these statements, we are currently using a test system (*i.e.*, the mouse) for routine carcinogenicity tests in which one is hard put to place much, if any, confidence. We can all agree that compounds that produce metastasising hepatic tumours in the mouse are carcinogens in the mouse, whether or not the observation can be extrapolated to other species. By contrast, compounds that are associated with nodular hyperplasia, or so called benign adenomas, pose a much greater problem. In these situations, detailed evaluation in other species is clearly needed before the observation can be accepted as an indication of the possible carcinogenic potential of a compound.

It is well known that potent enzyme inducers such as phenobarbital can produce hepatic nodules in the mouse. The enzyme systems induced are necessary for both activation and detoxification of various carcinogens, and changes in the enzymes, either by induction or inhibition, could increase or decrease the susceptibility of the mouse to chemical carcinogens or to oncogenic viruses. If one were to attempt to exclude all ancillary factors which may influence such susceptibility (*e.g.*, inherent susceptibility of the mouse; environmental factors), it would probably be necessary to conduct experiments essentially in a germ-free environment and use highly purified synthetic diets. Extrapolating these results to the real world situation would be even more difficult.

Most of us would probably agree that positive carcinogenicity data obtained in the mouse under standard laboratory conditions should not be accepted as definitive without validation in other species. The routine tests that are presently being conducted in the mouse could be considered as more an academic exercise in exploring a model than a scientific investigation capable of leading to valid, definitive conclusions about a compound. They can only provide clues that further investigations are needed.

In the light of information reviewed at this workshop, and in consideration of the various options available to us regarding carcinogenicity test systems, it would seem appropriate to seriously consider dropping the mouse as a biological test system for routine carcinogenicity testing, since it may be more misleading than helpful. Positive carcinogenicity data with a compound in any species can result in a serious stigma which can make the problem of sorting out the true situation practically impossible. For example, a short article published in 1963 (PAGET, 1963) indicated that one of a series of agents having beta-adrenergic blocking activity was carcinogenic in a special strain of mouse. Even though other tests in rats and dogs failed to show any evidence of a carcinogenic response in these species, regulatory reaction to the "positive" mouse data resulted in a moratorium on clinical research with beta-adrenergic blocking agents in the United States which persisted for more than two years and has only recently been rescinded. This situation was further confounded by the fact that the edict was applied to essentially all known beta-adrenergic blocking agents undergoing or about to undergo clinical investigation, and a whole pharmacologic class of agents was indicted without the usual regard for structure–activity relationships. Subsequent tests in several other strains of mice failed to show any evidence that the initial compound in question was uniformly carcinogenic in the mouse. Thus, a serious question is posed as to whether the risk to life involved in setting back research with beta-adrenergic blocking agents by two years was justified by the evidence of carcinogenicity which precipitated the regulatory action.

The scientific community is a heterogeneous group of individuals having sincere but diverse opinions, especially with respect to carcinogenesis. Certainly, we seem to be polarised in our views regarding the role of chemicals in this phenomenon. At one extreme are those individuals who feel that the only proved carcinogens are those which have been shown to be suspect by acceptable epidemiologic studies in man. At the other extreme are those individuals, and some rather highly vocal ones I might add, who take the rather simplistic view that a suggestive carcinogenic response in any species, at any dose, is absolute proof that the compound in question is a potential danger to man and should be immediately banned from the environment. One example of this philosophy is a situation in the U.S. that you know about, the so-called Delaney clause in the Food, Drug and Cosmetic Act, which initially was intended to be applied to food additives and other kinds of materials that might find their way into the food chain and be inadvertently ingested, or in which some other accidental exposure might occur. The rule is simply this, as I have just stated: any carcinogenic response, in any species, at any dose, immediately eliminates a compound from any further consideration. Thus, in the case of carcinogenesis, as opposed to other types of toxicologic investigations, the "all or nothing" rule applies. The dose–response concept is thus largely ignored, a situation that tends to violate the basic tenets of toxicology. Although such an interpretation has not yet been applied to drugs, it seems to be gradually gaining wider acceptance in various academic and governmental areas.

Those of us who must deal with real life situations in developing useful industrial, agricultural, and pharmaceutical chemicals feel that such an inflexible position poses a serious threat to further advances in the use of chemicals. Certainly, it is not suggested that we should assume a cavalier attitude by exposing mankind to a carcinogen or any other harmful agent, but it still remains that our test systems are imperfect, and that data developed in such systems should be given the most careful scrutiny before a potentially useful compound is relegated to oblivion. We know, of course, that emotion and a general fear of the unknown commands sympathetic ears in many regulatory and governing bodies around the world. It is unfortunate, however, that the very test systems that elicit these problems are themselves incapable of providing information upon which sound decisions can be made to resolve them. It seems to me that of the widely used test systems that are notably imperfect in this regard, the mouse probably should head the list.

Because of the economy, availability and a host of other factors, however, it is likely that the mouse will continue to be used as a major species for carcinogenicity testing, at least until a more predictive alternate test system can be established. Thus it seems appropriate that we consider various experimental alternatives which might accommodate the mouse despite the capricious nature of the species. It could be argued that the exquisite sensitivity of the mouse liver to a variety of chemical agents justifies the use of the species as a simple primary screen. If appropriate testing in other species should indicate that a carcinogenic response occurs only in the mouse, however, and then only in one sex, or at high doses, a very low level of probability should be assigned to that compound with respect to its carcinogenic potential. A carcinogenic response in the mouse liver alone, in the absence of positive data in other species, should be taken to indicate only that the test compound is carcinogenic in the mouse, and not in other untested species, including man.

Recently, I had an opportunity to participate as a member of a joint committee of the U.S. Food and Drug Administration and the Pharmaceutical Manufacturers Association charged with the task of developing guidelines for carcinogenicity tests. In these deliberations a great deal of thought was given to the choice of species for such tests. The capricious nature of the mouse in carcinogenicity and other types of safety testing was recognized; however, it was listed as an acceptable species primarily because other choices were either limited or unavailable. Two species were suggested, *i.e.*, rat and mouse, although selection was left largely to the discretion of the investigator.

In developing information upon which to assign levels of "relative safety" or "risk factors", a statistical formula such as that proposed by MANTEL AND BYRAN (1961) might be considered. These authors suggest that some estimate of a dose of a given agent can be devised which could be considered "virtually safe". This assumes, of course, that one first defines some arbitrary level of permissible risk, no matter how small, rather than insisting on absolute safety which is, of course, unobtainable. The point of interest is that since direct observations cannot be made which establish unequivocally that the risk at some dose is clearly low, indirect conservative procedures for the determination of low risk levels become necessary.

MANTEL AND BYRAN (1961) state, "Absolute safety can never be unquestionably demonstrated experimentally. Rather, experimental results can be used only to establish limits on the risk involved. With the specification of some level of risk, no matter how small, the possibility of determining whether or not that risk is exceeded opens. We may, for example, assume that a risk of 1/100 million is so low as to constitute "virtual safety." Other arbitrary definitions of "virtual safety" may be employed as conditions require.".

"In principle, one could use an experimental protocol sufficiently large to demonstrate that "virtual safety" obtained. For this purpose it must be realised that an observed outcome of no tumours among 100 million treated mice does not necessarily demonstrate clearly that treatment was either absolutely or virtually safe. This outcome could arise with a probability that the risk was under 1 percent, even if the risk involved were as high as 4.6/100 million. It would in fact require a total of some 460 million tumour-free mice to demonstrate at the 99 percent assurance level that "virtual safety" obtained. Similarly, tumour-free results for 10 000 mice would only indicate that the risk was less than 1/2200 and it would require tumour-free results in a total of some 450 mice to establish with high probability that the risk was under 1 percent."

Such astronomical figures required for direct observation tend to stagger the imagination. However, the statistical formula devised by these investigators is based on the assumption that the relationship observed between tumour occurrence and dose at the levels tested will continue to apply in the regions to which extrapolation is being made, in which situation studies of feasible size can be used. It is apparent, of course, that the first requirement for such a statistical formula is that the carcinogenic dose be defined, and that the dose–response concept be accepted for carcinogenicity evaluation as it is for other types of toxicologic investigations. I think we can agree that in the present state of the art the use of the mouse for such purposes would pose a considerable problem. In the absence of other workable systems, however, such an approach might be considered in arriving at decisions regarding "relative safety" or "risk factors".

Recently in the U.S. the available carcinogenic data on 14 compounds which were considered to be known or suspected carcinogens in man were screened by scientists of the National Institute of Occupational Safety and Health (NIOSH). The purpose of the review was to make recommendations regarding the handling and use of these substances in industrial and research settings. Since this exercise represents an attempt on the part of knowledgeable individuals to extrapolate experimental data to man, and cites the basis for conclusions that were drawn, a brief discussion of these data would appear to be pertinent.

Certain data on six compounds considered to be carcinogenic in man are shown in Tables I–VI, primarily to indicate the role, if any, of the mouse. As can be seen from these data, the organ response reported for mouse and man was similar for only 3 of the 6 compounds (*i.e.* similar with chloromethyl methyl ether (CMME), bis(chloromethyl) ether (BCME) and 4-aminodiphenyl (4-ADP); dissimilar with benzidine, α-naphthylamine (1-NA) and β-naphthylamine (2-NA). The data also reflect the differences or similarities in other species used in these investigations.

SUMMARY

In this workshop we have examined in detail the fundamental problem of the response of the mouse liver to chemical agents. Objective criteria have not been defined that would clearly indicate whether the mouse liver accurately reflects the general carcinogenicity of a compound. The utility of the mouse for purposes of routine screening of chemicals for carcinogenic potential is, therefore, highly questionable. For these reasons, it is suggested that strong consideration be given to deleting the mouse as a routine test animal for such purposes, although the species should definitely be retained as a useful system for studies in experimental carcinogenesis. Development of other acceptable test systems is an urgent need.

A reliable procedure for assigning levels of significance (*i.e.* relative safety, risk factor) to carcinogenic responses should be developed. It is suggested that such a system might well incorporate as one facet the statistical treatment of data such as that proposed by MANTEL AND BYRAN (1961). This would require that a carcinogenic dose be defined, and that the dose–response concept be accepted for carcinogenicity evaluation as it is for other types of toxicological investigations.

ACKNOWLEDGEMENTS

The suggestions and assistance of R. CARLSON, R. HANNAH, W. KNAPP, F. PLETZ, R. POWELL, J. SWENBERG AND M. WEINER in preparation of this report are gratefully acknowledged.

TABLE I

BENZIDINE

Species	Route	Dose/duration	Target organ(s)	Comment
Rat	sc	15 mg/wk (lifetime)	Liver (M)	Tumours in males only
	sc	300 mg/6 months	Liver	
			Ear	
			Injection site	
	oral	5 mg × 10 (q 3 days)	Mammary gland	
	vapour	27 mg/20 months	WBC (leukaemia)	
			Mammary gland	Tumours in males and
			Liver	females
Dog	diet	325 g in 5 yrs	Bladder	1 carcinoma in 7 dogs
Monkey	sc	50–200 mg/wk		
		(duration N.S.)[a]		No carcinogenic effect
Rabbit	sc	75–100 mg/wk		
		(duration N.S.)[a]		No carcinogenic effect
Mouse	sc	6 mg/wk 15–28 months	Liver	
Hamster	diet	0.1% lifetime	Liver	
			Biliary sys.	
Man	N.S.[a]	Occupational		
		exposure	Bladder	Interpretation complicated
			Kidney	by concomitant exposure
			Pancreas	to other known carcinogens

[a] Not stated.

(Data excerpted from NIOSH Report, July, 1973)

TABLE II

ALPHA-NAPHTHYLAMINE (1-NA)

Species	Route	Dose/duration	Target organ(s)
Mouse	Drinking water	100 mg/l (duration N.S.)[a]	None reported
	oral	250 mg (single dose)	None reported
Rabbit	ip	150 mg/wk (1-0.5 yr)	
Man	Occupational exposure	(duration N.S.)[a]	Bladder

Note: 1-NA is frequently contaminated with 2-NA, a known carcinogen.
[a] Not stated.
(Data excerpted from NIOSH Report, June, 1973)

TABLE III

BETA-NAPHTHYLAMINE (2-NA)

Species	Route	Dose	Target organ(s)
Dog	sc and diet	variable	Bladder
	oral	310 g total	Bladder
	oral	1000–2000 mg/wk	Bladder
Rat	oral	0.067% in diet	Bladder
			Liver
			Lung
	ip	100 mg/kg/wk	Abdomen (injection site)
			Salivary gland
Mouse	sc	3 g/50 wk	Liver
Monkey	oral	6.25–400 mg/kg	Bladder
Hamster	oral	1% in diet	Bladder
Man	Occupational exposure	Unknown	Bladder

(Data excerpted from NIOSH Report, July, 1973)

TABLE IV

CHLOROMETHYL METHYL ETHER (CMME)

Species	Route	Dose/duration	Target organ(s)	Comment
Mouse	topical	6 mg/wk (42 wk)	See comment	Incomplete carcinogen
	sc	125 ml/kg (single)	See comment	Some BCME contaminant
	vapour	2 ppm (10 exposures)	Lung	Carcinogenicity not definitely established because of contamination with BCME.
	sc	300 μg/wk (26 wk)	Injection site	
Rat	sc	1-3 mg (3-4 times/month)	Injection site	Palpable lesions; not defined as malignancies.
	topical 1000 and 100 μg	(duration N.S.)[a]	Application site	Possible "irritating agent" (phorbol ester promoting agent).
	sc	3 mg (duration N.S.)[a]	Injection site	
Man	Occupational exposure	Unknown (1–14 yrs)	Lung	High incidence of oat cell carcinoma. *Note:* CMME hydrolized to MeOH + HCOH + HCl which recombines to BCME spontaneously.

[a] Not stated.
(Data excerpted from NIOSH Report. May, 1973)

TABLE V

BIS(CHLOROMETHYL) ETHER (BCME)

Species	Route	Dose/duration	Target organ(s)	Comment
Mouse	topical	6 mg/wk (50 wk)	Application site	
	sc	12.5 ml/kg (single dose)	Lung	
	vapour	1 ppm (82 days)	Lung	Only slightly higher tumor incidence in treated over control.
Rat	parenteral	9 mg/mo (9 months)	Injection site	
	vapour	0.1 ppm (101 exposure)	Lung Nose	
Man	vapour	Unknown	Lung	Increased incidence of oat cell carcinoma.

(Data excerpted from NIOSH Report, June, 1973)

TABLE VI

4-AMINODIPHENYL (4-ADP)

Species	Route	Dose/duration	Target organ(s)	Comment
Dog	oral	Variable	Bladder	
	oral	0.9 g/wk (34 mo)	Bladder	
	oral	0.5 g/wk (3 yr)	Bladder	
	oral	50 mg/kg (single dose)		No tumours during 5 years observation
Rat	sc	N.S.[a]	Liver Intestine Mammary gland	
Rabbit	oral	Limit of tolerance	Bladder	
Mouse	oral	38 mg/9 months (2 × wk)	Bladder	
	oral	1.5 mg/wk (× 5 wk)	Liver Bladder	
	sc	200 mg (single dose)	Liver	Increased incidence of hepatomas; 19/20 males; 4/23 females
Man	Occupational exposure	Unknown	Bladder	High incidence of bladder tumours

[a] Not stated.
(Data excerpted from NIOSH Report, June, 1973)

REFERENCES

MANTEL, N., AND BYRAN, W. R. (1961) "Safety" Testing of Carcinogenic Agents. *J. Natl. Cancer Inst.*, 27: 455-470.
PAGET, G. E. (1963) Carcinogenic Action of Pronethalol. *Brit. Med. J.*, 2: 1266-1267.

DISCUSSION

P. M. NEWBERNE. It might be of interest to those of you that do not know how the information in the NIOSH report is developed, to outline the procedure. The usual approach is to have a list of recommendations printed in the Federal Register so that the recommendations may be reviewed by anybody interested and a time limit is set for this response. It is germain to what we are considering here that the language is such that although they chose the limited number of compounds indicated by Dr. J. W. NEWBERNE, at any time the list can be added to by just printing it in the Federal Register. This was primarily aimed at manufacturing companies making compounds which may be carcinogenic or anything that could be considered a carcinogen, but it very quickly drew in everybody who had used carcinogens. As a result of this it is going to become increasingly difficult to do basic research with carcinogens. Many research labs are trying to determine how they are going to meet the requirements that are very specifically set forth. In essence, it is going to be very close to a germ-free type of operation. If this is really enforced we may not be doing much research for a number of years in the field of carcinogenesis. Nobody will argue with the need to be extremely careful with carcinogens but I think by and large most laboratories have been.

174

BUTLER. Were all the compounds considered to be carcinogenic in man before being tested in animals?

J. W. NEWBERNE. Not necessarily in that order. The epidemiological studies took a long time and during that period some testing was done. When the decision was made on man, some data in other species were available.

ROE. When considering the predictive value of the mouse and the occurrence of liver neoplasms in mice resulting from their exposure to chemical agents, it is necessary to consider the comprehensive review on this subject by TOMATIS et al. (1973). The fact that they gave their paper a misleading title and reached a number of unjustifiable conclusions is dwarfed by the comprehensiveness of their coverage of the published literature. All of us are indebted to them for this.

The title of the review was *The Predictive Value of Mouse Liver Tumour Induction in Carcinogenicity Testing—a Literature Survey* and in it they refer to data on 58 chemical substances. About half of these were recognised as potent carcinogens for other animal species *before* any investigator had the temerity to test them for activity in the mouse. Thus the "discovery" that these substances increased the incidence of liver tumours in mice had no *predictive* value as far as carcinogenicity for other species and tissues was concerned, since these activities were already known.

The review reminded me of a paper published in 1968 of which I was a co-author [GORROD et al. (1968) *J. Natl. Cancer Inst.*, 41: 403]. In that paper we reported that 4-aminobiphenyl given at birth increased the incidence of liver-cell tumours in Swiss mice killed at one year from 3/41 in untreated males to 19/20 in treated males and from 0/43 in untreated females to 4/23 in treated females. Tumours were usually multiple in mice that bore them. There was no increased incidence of tumours of other sites. Before we carried out our tests 4-aminobiphenyl had been reported as carcinogenic for adult mice, rats, dogs, rabbits and man. TOMATIS et al. (1973), however, overlooked the fact that, in the same study, we also found 3 hydroxylated derivatives of 4-aminobiphenyl to have similar, though slightly less marked, effects on liver tumour incidence. These were 4-amino-3-hydroxybiphenyl (I), 4-hydroxyaminobiphenyl (II), and 4-amino-4'-hydroxybiphenyl (III). Attempts to produce bladder tumours in mice by the implantation of intravesical pellets containing I were successful but pellets containing II or III gave negative results [BONSER et al. (1963) *Brit. J. Cancer*, 17: 127; Clayson et al. (1958) *Brit. J. Cancer*, 12: 222; Boyland et al. (1964) *Brit. J. Cancer*, 18: 575]. No tumours arose in rats fed a diet containing I [Miller et al. (1956) *Cancer Res.*, 16: 525].

However, my concern about the conclusions drawn by TOMATIS et al., is more serious and more fundamental than a mere quibble about the meaning of "predictive value", or than a worry that they have overlooked important facts in the papers they reviewed. I believe it to be important to define the word "induction" in the context of the occurrence of neoplasms in animals that have been exposed to a test chemical or other stimulus. In so far as all the kinds of neoplasm seen in response to exposure to chemical agents also arise, albeit in some cases only rarely, in unexposed animals, it is possible to argue that carcinogenesis is never anything more than enhancement of a naturally occurring phenomenon. "Spontaneously" occurring neoplasms may result from the exposure of animals to tumour-inducing agents present in the background "environment". Increased incidence of neoplasms of the same kinds in response to a test chemical may occur: *(i)* If the test chemical induces additional neoplasms; *(ii)* If the chemical enhances the effect of tumour inducers present in the background environment.

This distinction might be of only academic interest if the test animal is man. A factory owner might be just as liable for damages if one of his employees developed cancer as a result of exposure to a co-carcinogen at work as he would be if exposure was to a carcinogen. The distinction becomes less academic as the possible hazard to man becomes more theoretical. The purpose of screening chemicals for carcinogenicity is to predict carcinogenic risk to man and not simply to try to divide substances into two categories: carcinogens and non-carcinogens. The result of a single animal test, whether negative or positive, is liable to be grossly misleading. Confidence in the prediction that exposure to a substance is likely to constitute or not to constitute a cancer hazard for man increases as information becomes available from studies conducted under a range of conditions and in a range of species. If positive results from only one study are available, confidence that they are predictive of hazard for man is higher if the kind or kinds of tumour found in excess incidence occur only rarely in unexposed animals. Under these circumstances common sense dictates that the "extra" tumours are more likely to have been the result of induction by the test chemical than of enhancement of the activity of a background carcinogen. By contrast, a mere increase in the incidence of a commonly occurring phenomenon is difficult to interpret, especially where it is already known that a wide variety of other, non-specific, factors may influence the incidence of the same phenomenon. This, I would suggest, is the position when the only evidence that a substance is a carcinogen is that exposure to it results in an increased incidence of liver-cell adenomas and adenocarcinomas in a strain of mice in which tumours of the same kind occur spontaneously in high incidence.

When I first used the term background environment I surrounded the word "environment" by inverted commas. It may be that vertically transmissible viruses as well as genetic factors help to determine high risk of spontaneous liver tumour development. For the sake of simplicity I include this possibility within the broad term "environment".

TOMATIS *et al.* (1973) restricted their view to neoplasms of liver-parenchymal-cell origin, but some of the 58 substances they listed also produced primary liver tumours of other kinds. The types of tumour which occur spontaneously in high incidence in some strains of mice are adenomas and adenocarcinomas of parenchymal-cell origin. Tumours of intra-hepatic bile duct origin and of vascular origin occur spontaneously only rarely by comparison. It would be reasonable, therefore, to be more concerned about a chemical that gave rise to cholangiomatous and angiomatous tumours of the liver as well as to tumours of parenchymal-cell origin than about one that did no more than increase the incidence of parenchymal-cell tumours.

REUBER. This is really a very difficult field in which to make any sense. Most people to whom I have talked feel that before you can make any safe extrapolation between any experimental animal and man, it is necessary to show that the metabolism is similar in both man and the test species, but I am uncertain how realistic this is. I do not think anybody is saying that following a carcinogenicity test in the mouse or rat that one can draw any conclusion for man. All we are saying is that at the moment the means that we have chosen to decide whether a chemical is harmful is a test in animals, and, if it is harmful to animals, we conclude that it is a harmful substance. There may be more sensible ways of making comparisons between man and animals than metabolic studies, but I do not think that anybody has attempted to do this. I think that people are taking the easy way out saying we cannot do it with the mouse. If we use the mouse and rat and demonstrate a liver carcinoma, there is no reason at all that I can think of that, if man were to get the same compound, we should consider that the site at which neoplasia might develop in man would also be the liver. It is just as reasonable to assume that cancer could develop at another site.

I do not know why we should come to a conclusion that an experimental animal is useful or not. This is something each laboratory must decide for themselves. If they are not required to use mouse, then another species may be used. Until one is told to use a specific species, it is up to each investigator to decide.

ROE. May I ask if you have a positive test in an animal and did metabolic studies finding that man and the animal metabolised the compounds differently, would you be less worried about the risk to man? If a test gave a negative response in animals, and it was then found that man metabolised the compound in a different way, would you regard this as negative evidence of safety?

REUBER. I do not know as I am not qualified to assess this.

GRASSO. We have given some thought to this at BIBRA and we have wondered whether similarity in metabolism is meaningful as we do not know the identity of the carcinogenic metabolite. We consider that if we get a positive result in a rat or mouse and then if possible metabolic work in man, we would then choose a species which metabolises the compound as man. This may be a step nearer selecting the correct species.

P. M. NEWBERNE. The tendency to go to more and more metabolic studies is excellent. On the other hand, the more that is done seemingly the less we know what is of significance. This is reflected in the two cases of benzidine and β-naphthylamine. What is of concern is the bladder cancer and neither the rat nor the mouse would be a good predictor of this.

J. W. NEWBERNE. On benzidine, the rat, dog, rabbit and mouse all have the same major metabolite of the 3-hydroxybenzidine.

GRASSO. What is the value of identifying a major metabolite? I would presume that if a substance appears in the urine it means that it has been inactivated in some way. What we want to know is what is the carcinogenic intermediate and this is extremely difficult.

J. W. NEWBERNE. I agree entirely. The problem is that one tends to rank metabolites in the order in which they occur. In this connection if one comes back to the problem of extrapolating to man, any toxicological data are analogous to this. An interesting example is the problem of cataracts in animals and man. An experimental drug was found to cause cataracts in rats and dogs but not monkeys. There was a major attempt to determine in the dog which metabolite, if any, or the parent compound was causing the cataract. The only consistent finding was cataracts. There were at least five metabolites in the rat and dog for example which did not occur in man and major differences also between monkeys and man with no correlation possible between drug metabolism and cataract formation [SMITH et al. (1973) J. Int. Drug Res., 1: 489]. It is very difficult to bring metabolism into this. When one looks at the problem of metabolism, there are enormous differences in body burdens between the mouse and man and any other animal, even though they might have produced the same metabolites. The assessment of the final effect becomes a very difficult matter. Over and above the identity of the metabolites, it is necessary to know if they bind to cell constituents and stay in situ, or whether they are freely mobile throughout the animal.

ROE. We are all over-simplifying the matter. When a compound is being assessed on its merits, one takes into account metabolic data, absorption, target species, pharmacokinetic studies among others. I do not think that rules can be made to cover this. A well-functioning regulatory body should look at all this information. One question is crucial. Do you regard the mouse liver tumour system as a very sensitive system, a too sensitive system, for revealing carcinogenicity or do you regard it as a system picking up some carcinogens but also some non-carcinogens and some non-specific factors as co-carcinogens? The latter is my view. On the basis of the present knowledge I find it a misleading system for the very reason that no expert we have listened to has controlled all the factors which may influence the incidence of tumours. If all these factors were controlled, one might then have a sensitive test. However, a test of very great sensitivity may still be misleading because it reveals hazards which are not really hazards.

BUTLER. I think that the points raised by Dr. ROE are the crucial ones for us. Is the mouse liver system misleading or too sensitive? I am uncertain on what Dr. REUBER was basing his remarks: whether it is just the general premise that man and mouse are both mammals and therefore react in the same way in producing the same lesions, or whether you consider that there is experimental evidence for similarity or whether it is based on an assessment of the pathology.

REUBER. I don't think I said any of those things. We have just chosen a means to test something. Therefore that is what we use. I would go further to say that if experimental tumours in animals and man look alike and behave alike biologically, I think that they are comparable lesions. The main benefit we get from this is that if we want to study a particular aspect such as histogenesis of a particular carcinoma, we look for a model that has the same characteristics that one finds in man.

THORPE. What you are saying is highly commendable and is the attitude of the cancer research worker who seeks to unravel the mechanisms of carcinogenesis. If I may comment on Dr. ROE's conclusion that the mouse liver tumour system is misleading, I think that if at first sight one does not look at mechanisms of interaction, it can be very misleading. From what we have heard this week, there are a great many factors which we all agree are not carcinogenic but which can radically modify the number, time of appearance and indeed the morphology of the lesions which do appear. In essence, it may be an expression of our ignorance that we rely on the experimental pathologist to come up with a definitive answer as to whether a compound is likely or not to be carcinogenic to man. If you have a response such as we have seen in mouse liver, the next step should be to look at the human epidemiology if it exists as well as the information derived from biochemists, of metabolic studies. These metabolic studies on their own give no definitive answers and it is no comfort to say that the rodent and man have the same metabolic profiles. What one is concerned about is the interaction of the active species and biological macromolecules, in other words, the mechanism of induction. Faced as we are in many cases not having these data, one has to seek the evidence for established compounds. This has been done in the case of phenobarbitone. In three studies it has been shown to induce nodules in the mouse liver which in our laboratory are associated with metastases and successful transplantation. This evidence is something which we must take note of. CLEMMESEN [(1974) *Lancet*, ii: 705] looked at the necropsy data of a population of long-term epileptics who had been treated with phenobarbitone and other anti-convulsants. The total neoplastic spectrum in these patients was no different than that of control groups except for tumours of the central nervous system, as was expected. He concluded that, from his information, these compounds are not carcinogenic for man. Lastly, if you start with a novel compound and the response is that mouse liver nodules are increased, in the absence of positive data from other species it would be short-sighted to abandon that compound immediately. Rather than call the mouse misleading we should consider the result as a little man with a red flag say, "here is a possible problem which warrants looking at in depth. Don't throw away the compound and don't advance too quickly".

ROE. I think we are all aware that, in general, compounds which have been tested and given equivocal results suffer more at the hands of regulatory authorities than similar substances which have not been tested. If data are submitted which happens to include a solitary positive finding, *e.g.* that the incidence of liver tumours in mice is increased, it is bad luck to have chosen a strain of mouse that is particularly sensitive. The problem is that in some regulatory systems this pushes a compound from the non-banned into the banned category. The repercussions of this sort of decision made on this kind of data are well-known. It means that companies draw back from doing unnecessary testing, unnecessary as determined by it not being a strict requirement. It might be very sensible to do the test, but their advisors will tell you that you do this at your peril as you might get a result which is difficult to interpret. Somebody in a regulatory authority will choose to interpret it as a bad thing. This is counterproductive. If I look at a whole range of substances, I do not have a nil suspicion about any. As you get information your suspicion either increases or decreases. If your only evidence of a positive effect is an increased incidence of liver tumours in the mouse, this only pushes my suspicion up a little. Whereas other people take an entirely different view; it pushes their suspicion right up to the top through the level at which you ban the compound. This is a hyper-reactive response and, on the basis of the information we have, is entirely illogical.

P. M. NEWBERNE. This is a key point. If an experiment is done and reported it has to be dealt with. For that reason, many things are not looked at any more than they have to be. They will only be looked at when it is required.

Chapter 10

Summary

The following comments were invited by the Chairman of the meeting at the last session and are taken from the recordings of the meeting and from notes submitted by the speakers.

Editors.

H. G. Grice. The papers and discussions of the meetings this week have strengthened my views that from a regulatory standpoint the use of mouse strains with a high spontaneous incidence of hepatic tumours for routine carcinogenicity testing is undesirable.

I would prefer not to have to evaluate submissions containing information on mouse hepatic tumours with two possible exceptions. In both cases it is assumed that information would be available on a second species:

(1) In those instances in which there was no statistical difference in the incidence of hepatic neoplasms between treated and control groups (suggesting the compound might not be carcinogenic).

(2) In those instances in which there was a highly significant dose-related increase in the incidence of hepatic neoplasms in the treated groups along with additional information on all factors that are known to alter the incidence of tumours in the strain used.

Unfortunately, my experience has been that the latter type of information is not available. Often the difference in incidence of hepatic neoplasms between treated and control animals is not great and there is no good dose–response relationship. The statisticians have to resort to unusually refined techniques to show differences. In addition information is usually lacking on dietary, environmental and physical factors that are known to alter the spontaneous incidence of the tumours, *i.e.* detailed information on food consumption, food utilization, viral status of the host, effects of the test compound on the immune status of the host and so on. Even if we had all this information, we would still be left with the lingering doubt that some combination of these factors was responsible for an increased incidence.

It is apparent that before strains of mice with a spontaneous incidence of hepatic tumours can be considered as a suitable test species in routine carcinogenicity testing, considerable work will have to be done to provide a better understanding of the aetiology and pathogenesis of the tumours. Included in studies that might be undertaken to gain this understanding are the following:

(1) Effects of varying dietary constituents including fatty acids and fatty acid isomers.

(2) Variations in environmental temperature including slight increase or decrease (*e.g.* $72 \pm 5°$) as well as heat or cold stress.

(3) Other forms of environmental stress—*i.e.* number of animals per cage, type of caging.

(4) Effects of an altered immune system.

(5) Viral studies—viruses as aetiologic agents.

(6) Comparative morphometric analysis of A and B lesions—spontaneous and induced as well as comparative studies of hypertrophic cells in young mice (induced) and old animals (control lesions). Biochemical and histochemical studies should be run concurrently with morphometric studies.

(7) Cell kinetic studies to determine cell turn-over rates in the various lesions and control or normal liver.

And perhaps for someone who has an inexhaustable budget and unlimited time, studies on the effect of combinations of the above factors in altering the spontaneous incidence.

It has been suggested that the mouse served a useful purpose as a screen for potential carcinogens. Perhaps it should be used for this purpose for the time being. We have recently reviewed other short-term tests that may have application for this purpose [Stoltze *et al.* (1974) *J. Toxicol. appl. Pharmacol.*, 29: 157]. U.S. National Cancer Institute studies designed to assess several of the short-term tests will hopefully provide information concerning the suitability and reliability of these tests as screens for carcinogens.

As far as a second suitable species for routine carcinogenicity testing is concerned, the hamster may hold some promise in this regard. It is being used successfully for this purpose at the Eppley Institute in Omaha and several of the participants at this meeting have indicated that they are considering the hamster. We have studies underway in our laboratory to determine the suitability of the hamster for our particular purposes in carcinogenicity testing.

G. LAQUEUR. In summarizing the impressions I have had of this workshop on the classification and biology of nodules in the liver of mice, I should first of all cite the two excellent papers presented by Dr. GRASSO and Dr. GELLATLY. Both of these presentations presented extensive reviews of the literature on the incidence of liver nodules as influenced by genetic factors (Dr. GRASSO) and by a broad spectrum of environmental factors among which nutrition and particularly the lipids assumed an important role (Dr. GELLATLY). In spite of these important discussions so well presented, the aetiology and pathogenesis of these liver nodules as well as their biologic significance have largely remained unresolved. The difficulties are increasing when this system is used in analysing possible carcinogenicity of substances to be tested by superimposing them upon the poorly understood system.

My personal recommendation would be for those interested in utilizing liver nodules or tumours in mice to go back to the laboratory and learn more about these "spontaneous" lesions in the liver of mice. I think we can all agree that "spontaneous" or "background" tumours are words substituted for things we do not as yet know or know only poorly or in part. Such an effort, the goal of which is to really understand liver tumours in mice, should preferably be a joint effort among competent scientists representing various disciplines. They should include virologists, nutritionists, biochemists, geneticists, and immunologists, in addition to morphologists and cell biologists.

Until the "spontaneous" hepatic nodules and tumours in mice are better understood, I would adhere to the rule of classifying these liver nodules according to the general principles of pathology in benign and malignant tumours. Local invasiveness and distant metastases are evidence of malignancy in this system, a fact with which a majority of us would agree. Local invasiveness in the absence of demonstrated metastases I also would take as evidence of malignancy, particularly when associated with some pleomorphic or abnormal appearance of the cells composing the nodule. Whether transplantability of liver nodules *per se* is an indication for malignancy, as has been suggested in this workshop in a careful study, I am not ready to follow, although metastases from a successful transplant would strongly favour that the transplant had been obtained from a malignant primary cancer. In this connection, it would also be desirable therefore to include in the future studies investigations of the factors controlling and governing the mechanisms of metastasis in mice since transplantability studies are sometimes substituted for the frequent absence of metastases as indicators of the malignant nature of the primary lesion.

E. THORPE. The problem may be broken down into two questions: *(1)* The significance of liver nodules in the mouse; *(2)* The on-going debate about the diagnosis of the lesions we see.

All I would really like to say on this is that I do not think that the working division we used has misled anyone. I think it still works and I would like to emphasize two points: *(a)* it is obviously not exclusive of other lesions; I am sure at some stage all of us will have seen or may yet see a form of highly anaplastic liver carcinoma which bears no resemblance to the working classification we have used; *(b)* when one is working with compounds one must not forget that the compound itself has quite definite effects on the cytology of individual cells, both within the nodular growths and in the liver outside the nodules, usually showing a zonal distribution. This can in fact, not only provide a pitfall for the unwary, but must be taken into account when making judgements on the significance of certain cytological changes which are seen.

S. TAKAYAMA. Two points appear to arise from this meeting. Dr. BUTLER suggested that a distinction should be made between clinical diagnosis and diagnosis in an experimental animal. In many human cases, many fully developed malignant tumours are easy to diagnose even if small. In experimental work this is not so easy. In 1930 YAMAGIWA demonstrated that coal tar induced neoplastic lesions in the rabbit ear. However, everybody did not agree that the tumours were malignant in the absence of metastases. When the experiments were continued for 3 years, metastases were found.

Recently Dr. SUGIMURA induced stomach cancer with nitrosoguanidine, and in the initial reports again no metastases or local invasion were demonstrated. If we investigate the carcinogenicity of an unknown substance in rodents, it is necessary to demonstrate the presence of invasion and metastases and cellular atypism before diagnosing carcinoma.

The mouse is useful for testing for carcinogenicity, but the problems presented by variations in food, strain and conditions of care make it necessary to use another species as well, *i.e.* rat or hamster. The problems arise if we only get a positive result in the mouse. In Japan a food additive was shown to be mutagenic and carcinogenic in mice. But is this valid? If we use the mouse and a compound produces a malignant tumour, can this be extrapolated to man? This is a great problem that I do not know how to answer.

P. GRASSO. Three main items have been discussed at great depth at this meeting: *(1)* histological diagnosis; *(2)* the importance of transplantability; *(3)* value of the induction of liver tumours as an index of carcinogenicity.

(1) It appears to be well established that metastases are associated with one recognisable histological pattern of lesion with adenoid and papillary formation and with no other type. In my view, in spite of the fact that only between 2–10% have been shown to metastasise, I would consider such an architecture as highly suspicious and very probably an indication of malignancy in the absence of metastases. I would give my opinion as histological adenocarcinoma. This practice is followed in other species and other organs of the mouse, and I do not see why the mouse liver should be made an exception. When better techniques than histology are available for detecting metastasis, perhaps this view could be modified.

(2) I have no first-hand experience of transplantation but the works of REUBER and GELLATLY indicate to me that transplantation studies could confirm under certain conditions two important features: *(a)* autonomy and *(b)* the property of local invasion and ability to kill the host.

(3) An increase of liver tumour incidence over that of the controls in mice is not to my mind a valid index of carcinogenicity of a compound because of the multiplicity of factors involved. In my view the use of a strain with a high natural incidence further reduces the significance. On the whole, the mouse is better avoided in the choice of species for screening compounds for carcinogenicity.

M. GELLATLY. The problems in mouse liver which have been discussed at this meeting have been summarised and discussed by HIGGINSON AND SVOBODA (*Path. Ann.*, 1970) and illustrate that a similar problem exists in man. As a comparative pathologist concerned not only with neoplastic change but with the broad spectrum of tissue change associated with degenerative, inflammatory, reparative and neoplastic processes, I have to accept that there are variations in these tissue responses which produce different patterns of disease in different species. At the same time I am well aware that animal models of human disease are rare. Despite all these facts, I must also recognize that the basic components of certain fundamental processes such as inflammation are common to all mammals. In normal tissues the range of structural and functional properties is limited, but under certain circumstances new populations of cells may be induced. The range of properties possessed by these cells is still limited, but one new property, that of cell multiplication at a level greater than in the normal tissue, is acquired. But, it is not this multiplication *per se* which determines the biological characteristics of this new population, but the rate of multiplication. My opinion is that slow growth, homogenicity and a high degree of differentiation are characteristic of hyperplasia and many of Dr. THORPE's "A" lesions exhibit these. In contrast, in other nodules (Dr. THORPE's Type "B" lesion) there is evidence of a different cell population of variable structure and organisational pattern. Such a population may not possess the properties of invasion and metastasis, but the heterogenicity of such a population and the loss of structure differentiation within such lesions are in my opinion as a general pathologist and not as an oncologist, sufficient criteria on which to establish the diagnosis of carcinoma.

A last impression which has come from this workshop is that many environmental and dietary influences may affect nodule incidence and until more information is available on these subjects, then as has been said time and again, results obtained from the mouse liver must be regarded as no more than a guide to possible carcinogenic effects.

C. F. HOLLANDER. Most has been said but I would like to make two comments. I appreciate the open discussion which has not changed my opinion that the mouse is a useful tool in studying the mechanism of either carcinogenesis or non-neoplastic diseases. I totally agree with Dr. LAQUEUR's view that we need a better insight into the mechanism of the induction of liver lesions. Other better models may be devised to study the problems of the progression of hyperplasia into malignancy.

Secondly, although I am not an expert on testing, we should not entirely abandon the mouse in certain aspects of screening. I think that it can be used as "the man waving the red flag" and until we know more about the nature of this lesion, we should use such knowledge. We might, at a later stage, knowing more about the lesion and its pathogenesis, decide whether to abandon it or not.

F. J. C. ROE, I agree with many of the comments which have been made, in particular, those of Dr. GRICE and Dr. LAQUEUR. I think that there has been a significant shift of opinion about the useful-ness of the mouse and especially its liver tumours since about 1968. I had my great doubts about mouse as early as that and to me it is a relief to see the data on which to base these doubts appearing.

I see, looking to the future, that we have had a warning with the mouse. Perhaps because it has been inbred, even the strains we regard as outbred are relatively inbred, and because of our whole labora-tory exercise with the mouse we have ruined it. We have somehow bred into it undesirable charac-teristics which are making it not useful for testing purposes. We have become conscious of the importance of the quantity and quality of the diet in relation to the mouse. I feel that this is a warning that these same problems may, in fact, be important in other species and in other tests. We should not go away saying we will abandon the mouse. We would say what have we learnt from this whole exercise. Let's make sure we do not ruin the rat and hamster by inbreeding. When we undertake car-cinogenicity tests in rats and hamsters we do not ignore what we have learnt about dietary control which has been highlighted in the mouse. So it comes back to an in-depth approach to work and of, one would hope, for an in-depth approach on the part of the regulatory authorities who are on the receiving end.

M. D. REUBER. The real problem we have to solve when it comes to testing is to devise a model system where we can cut the time from 2 years to 12–18 months. The system should be one in which we can have carcinomas in any organs, but none in the controls. Not only would this solve our problems about spontaneous tumours, but help to reduce the time it takes to identify harmful compounds and reduce the cost. I think that this can be done.

J. W. NEWBERNE. I would like to add my plea for additional information. We are stumbling over our ignorance of basic changes. Since we do not know what they are, we say a lot about them but under-stand little. This gives one a helpless feeling. We would all like to find our way out of this jungle, so I would make a plea for more work. Hopefully a concerted effort always keeping in mind those things which we do need to attend to closely, will help to move it up the scale a little.

I have learnt a lot from the conference in bringing us up to date on the present state of the art of what we can expect the mouse to do for us.

ADRIANNE ROGERS. I agree with Dr. LAQUEUR that we will have to learn a great deal more about this system before it is of practical use. In studies of hepatic regeneration we found many differences be-tween the rat and the mouse and found the mouse to respond less consistently than the rat.

GLENYS JONES. I only have limited experience in this field, but I have learnt a great deal from the meet-ing. I still feel that we must remember that we can only make our decisions on the facts we have avail-able and even though I am prepared to accept that possibly the "B" lesions described by Dr. THORPE and us and accepted by most people at this meeting may eventually prove to be malignant car-cinomas, we must have that proof before this terminology is used widely in the literature.

W. H. BUTLER. I will not attempt to give any summary of what has been said, except to say that I am much clearer in my own mind of our ignorance. This is important if one wants to do something about it. I would wholeheartedly agree with Dr. LAQUEUR that what we have to do is study mechanism and then one may apply the information to testing if that is the end product. I would consider it an awful prospect if the sole reason we studied mechanism of induction of any lesion was to devise a suitable toxicological test. I do not consider that the only basis for studying mechanism.

When we started to get this meeting together, it was our intention to get varying opinions represent-ed. At least in that, I am sure you will agree, we succeeded. I would like to thank all of you for coming here and taking a week to sit and discuss as Dr. NEWBERNE and I realise that you are all extremely busy.

Appendix I

Variation of Histological Diagnosis of Mouse Liver Tumours by Pathologists

SHOZO TAKAYAMA

Cancer Institute, Department of Experimental Pathology,
1-37-1 Kami-Ikebukuro,
Toshima-Ku, Tokyo 170 (Japan)

Mouse liver has been used extensively in recent years for chemical carcinogenesis studies and for carcinogenicity tests (TOMATIS *et al.*, 1973), but there have been a few reports on the histological description of liver cell neoplasms in mice (ANDERVONT AND DUNN, 1952; TAKAYAMA, 1968; BUTLER, 1971; URAGUCHI *et al.*, 1972; TURUSOV *et al.*, 1973). Criteria for the histological diagnosis of mouse liver cell neoplasms differ with individual researchers. The term "hepatoma" was first used (YAMAGIWA, 1911) for malignant neoplasms arising from human liver parenchymal cells but, in the literature, both malignant and benign neoplasms have conventionally been described as hepatoma. Most of the published reports deal with neoplasms which are not invasive or metastasising.

In order to study the variation of histological diagnosis of mouse liver neoplasms, 43 cases of both spontaneous and induced liver neoplasms were distributed to 15 experimental pathologists in Japan, who were asked to submit their histological diagnosis. The results of their diagnoses are described herein.

Slide number, mouse strain and sex, preparation of dose and route, and duration of experiment are summarized in Table I.

Table II lists the histological diagnosis by each individual according to the Comments on Pathology in the "Reports and Recommendations of Subcommittee on Morphology, Epidemiology and Pathology", *Liver Cancer*, IARC Scientific Publications No. 1, 1971.

Out of a total of 43 cases, identical diagnosis was returned by all the pathologists on 5 cases, and their diagnosis varied with all the others.

TABLE I

Slide No.	Strain	Sex	Carcinogen	Preparation and dose	Route and site	Duration of experiment (days)
5	C3Hf/Bi	M	Spontaneous			466
6	C3Hf/Bi	M	Spontaneous			492
7	CBA-T_6T_6/H	M	NBU	35 days after birth, NBU given for 60 days, total dose 53 mg	p. o.	365
8	ICR/JCL	M	N-OH-FAA	25 μg/mouse 1×, newborn	s. c.	365
9	ICR/JCL	M	DMBA	30 μg/mouse 1×, newborn	s. c.	365
10	ICR/JCL	F	DEN	50 μg/g 1×, 2 wk after birth	s. c.	270
11	ICR/JCL	M	2,7-FAA	Within 16 h after birth	s. c.	365
12	ICR/JCL	M	DEN	50 μg/g 1×, within 16 h after birth	s. c.	270
13	ICR/JCL	F	Transplanted tumour	Induced by 2,7-FAA	s. c.	60
14	ICR/JCL	M	2,7-FAA	0.025% in food during foetal period and afterward	Trans-placental and p. o.	180
15	C3H	M	NBU	0.5 mg/0.1 ml in olive oil 1×, 3 days old	s. c.	365
16	ICR/JCL	M	CCl_4, NBU	10 mg NBU/mouse, preceded at 24 h by 50% (0.1 ml) CCl_4 in olive oil 1×	s. c. and p. o.	435
17	ICR/JCL	M	CCl_4, NBU	as above	as above	435
18	ICR/JCL	M	CCl_4, NBU	20 mg NBU/mouse, preceded at 24 h by 50% (0.1 ml) CCl_4 in olive oil	as above	435
19	dd	M	α-BHC, β-BHC	each 250 ppm in food for 24 wk	p. o.	150
20	dd	M	Kanechlor-500	500 ppm in food for 48 wk	p. o.	336
21	dd	M	Kanechlor-500	500 ppm in food for 48 wk	p. o.	336
22	dd	M	α-BHC	500 ppm in food for 56 wk	p. o.	392
23	dd	M	α-BHC	250 ppm in food for 90 wk	p. o.	630
24	ICR/JCL	M	α-BHC	660 ppm in food for 35 wk, total dose 1117 mg	p. o.	245
25	ICR/JCL	M	2,7-FAA, α-BHC	660 ppm α-BHC in food for 16 wk (total 445 mg), preceded by 250 ppm 2,7-FAA in food for 4 wk (total 34 mg)	p. o.	365
26	ICR/JCL	M	2,7-FAA, α-BHC	as above	p. o.	365
27	ICR/JCL	M	2,7-FAA	660 ppm α-BHC in food for 10 wk (total 325 mg), preceded by 250 ppm 2,7-FAA in food for 10 wk (total 86 mg)	p. o.	365

TABLE I *(continued)*

Slide No.	Strain	Sex	Carcinogen	Preparation and dose	Route and site	Duration of experiment (days)
28	DDD	M	Luteoskyrin	320 μg/day in food for the 1st month, followed by 160 μg/day for 9 months	p. o.	370
29	DDD	M	Luteoskyrin	as above	p. o.	360
30	DDD	F	N-OH-FAA	2.5 mg/day in food for 30 wk	p. o.	470
31	ICR/JCL	M	α-BHC	600 ppm/day in food for 20 wk	p. o.	182
32	C57BL/6	M	Cycasin	0.5 mg/g 1 wk after birth	s. c.	480
33	C57BL/6	M	Cycasin	as above	s. c.	480
34	C57BL/6	M	Cycasin	as above	s. c.	480
35	C57BL/6	M	Cycasin	0.5 mg/g 1 wk old	s. c.	480
39	DDD		DMN	100 ppm in food for 184 days (total 29.3 mg)	p. o.	184
40	DDD		DMN	0.15 mg/mouse 1 × /wk for 25 wk, total dose 3.75 mg	s. c.	189
41	DDD		DMN	as above	s. c.	225
42	SJL/J	M	DMN	0.15 mg/mouse 1 × /wk for 15 wk	s. c.	247
43	ICR/JCL	M	DMN	5 ppm in drinking water for 4 wk	p. o.	365
45	ICR/JCL	M	DMN	as above	p. o.	365
46	DDD	M	Spontaneous			563
47	DDD	F	Spontaneous			563
48	C57BL/6	F	Spontaneous			525
49	BRSUNT/N		Spontaneous			485
50	C3H/He × BRSUNT/N	M	Spontaneous			496
51	C3H/He × BRSUNT/N	M	Spontaneous			496
52	C3H/He × BRSUNT/N	M	Spontaneous			496

Abbreviations: α-BHC, benzenehexachloride, α-isomer; β-BHC, benzenehexachloride, β-isomer; Cycasin, methylazoxymethanol β-glucoside; DEN, *N*-nitrosodiethylamine; DMBA, dimethylbenzanthracene; DMN, *N*-nitrosodimethylamine; 2,7-FAA, *N,N'*-2,7-fluorenylenebisacetamide; NBU, *N*-nitrosobutylurea; *N*-OH-FAA, *N*-hydroxy-*N*-fluoren-2-yl acetamide.

TABLE II

HISTOLOGICAL DIAGNOSES OF MOUSE LIVER NEOPLASMS BY 15 PATHOLOGISTS

Pathologist / Slide No.	1	2	3	4	5	6	7	8	9	10	11	12	13	14	15
5	1	1	1	1	1	1	1	1	2	1	1	1	1	2	1
6	3	3	3	3	2	3	3	3	2	2	2	3	3	3	2
7	1	2	2	2	2	2	3	3	3	3	2	3	3	3	2
8	3	2	3	2	2	3		2	3	3	2	3	3	3	3
9	2	2	2	1	1	1	1	2	2	1	1	3	1	2	2
10	2	2	2	3	2	2	2	3	3	3	2	2	3	3	2
11	1	1	2	1	2	2	1	2	2	2	2	1	3	2	2
12	1	1	2	1	1	1	1	1	2	1	1	1	1	1	1
13	2	1	1	1	1	1	1	1	2	1	1	1	1	1	1
14	1	2	1	1	1	1	1	1		1	1	2	1	2	1
15	2	1	1	1	1	1	1	1	1	1	1	2	1	1	1
16	2	2	2	2	2	2	3	2	3	2	2	2	2	2	2
17	1	1	1	1	2	1	1	1	1	1	2	1	1	1	1
18	2	2	2	2	2	2	2	2	3	2	2	2	2	2	2
19	2	3	3	2	3	2	3	2	3	1	3	1	1	3	2
20	2	2	3	2	1	2	3	2	3	1	3	3	2	2	2
21	2	3	3		3	2	1	2	3	1	1	2	2	2	2
22	2	3	3	2	3	2	3	2	3	2	2	2	2	2	2
23	1	1	1	1	1	1	1	1	1	1	1	1	1	1	1
24	3	3	3	2	3	2	3	3	3	1	2	3	3	3	2
25	3	3	3	3	3	3	3	3	3	3	3	3	3	3	3
26	1	1	1	2	1	1	1	1	1	1	1	1	2'	1	2'
27	1	1	1	3	1	1	1	3	1	1	1	1	2'	1	2'
28	3	3	3	2	3	2	3	2	3	1	2	3	2	3	3
29	1	1	1	1	1	1	1	1	2	1	1	1	1	1	1
30	1	1	1	1	1	1	1	1	1	1	1	1	1	1	1
31	2	1	2	1	1	1	1	1	2	1	1	2	1	2	1
32	1	1	1	1	1	1	1	1	2	1	1	1	1	1	1
33	1	1	1	1	1	1	1	1	1	1	1	1	1	1	1
34	1	1	1	1	1	1	1	1	1	1	1	1	1	1	1
35	2	1	1	1	1	1	1	1	1	1	1	1	2	1	1
39	1'	1'	2'	1'	2'	2'	2'	2'		2'	2'	1'	2'	1'	1'
40	1'	1'	2'	1'	2'	2'	2'	2'		2'	2'	1'	2'	1'	1'
41	1'	1'	1'	1'	2'	1'	2'	2'		2'	1'	1'	2'	1'	2'
42	1'	1'	2'	1'	2'	2'	2'	2'		2'	1'	1'	2'	1'	1'
43	1'	2' + 2	2'	2	2'	2'	2'	2'		2'	2'	2'	2' + 2	1'	1
45	1'	2'	2'	3'	2'	2'	1	2'	3	1	2'	2'	2'	1'	1
46	1'	2'	2'	2'	2'	2'	2'	2'		2'	2'	2'	2'	1'	2'
47	3	3	2	3	2	2	2	3	3	2	2	2	3	3	3
49	2	3	2	3	2	2	2	3	3	2	2	2	3	2	2
50	1	3	2	3	2	3	3	2	3	2	2	3	3	3	3
51	1	1	1	1	1	1	1	1	1	1	1	1	1	2	1
52	2	1	2	1	1	1	1	1	2	1	1	1	1	2	1

Explanation of figures:
1, Liver cell carcinoma.
2, Liver cell adenoma.
3, Hyperplastic nodule.
1', Haemangioendothelial sarcoma.
2', Haemangioma.
3', Hyperplasia of endothelial cell.

REFERENCES

ANDERVONT, H. B., AND DUNN, T. B. (1952) Transplantation of spontaneous and induced hepatomas in inbred mice. *J. Natl. Cancer Inst.*, 13: 455.

BUTLER, W. H. (1971) Pathology of liver cancer in experimental animals. In: *Liver Cancer*, IARC Scientific Publications No. 1, pp. 30–41. International Agency for Research on Cancer, Lyon, France.

TAKAYAMA, S. (1968) Induction of transplantable liver tumors in DBF$_1$ mice after oral administration of *N,N'*-2,7-fluorenylenebis-acetamide. *J. Natl. Cancer Inst.*, 40: 629.

TOMATIS, L., PARTENSKY, C., AND MONTESANO, R. (1973) The predictive value of mouse liver tumour induction in carcinogenicity testing—A literature survey. *Int. J. Cancer*, 12: 1.

TURUSOV, V. S., DERINGER, M. K., DUNN, T. B., AND STEWART, H. L. (1973) Malignant mouse-liver tumors resembling human hepatoblastomas. *J. Natl. Cancer Inst.*, 51: 1689.

URAGUCHI, K., SAITO, M., NOGUCHI, Y., TAKAHASHI, K., ENOMOTO, M., AND TATSUNO, T. (1972) Chronic toxicity and carcinogenicity in mice of the purified mycotoxins, luteoskyrin and cyclo-chlorotine. *Food Cosmet. Toxicol.*, 10: 193.

YAMAGIWA, K. (1911) *Arch. Path. Anat. Phys.*, 206: 437. Cited by YOSHIDA, T. (1944) *Carcinogenesis*, p. 89. Nippon Ishoshippan, Tokyo (in Japanese).

Subject Index

194